Advances in Treatment of Bipolar Disorder

Review of Psychiatry Series
John M. Oldham, M.D., M.S.
Michelle B. Riba, M.D., M.S.
Series Editors

Advances in Treatment of Bipolar Disorder

EDITED BY

Terence A. Ketter, M.D.

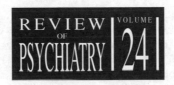

No. 3

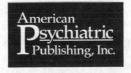

Washington, DC
London, England

Manufactured in the United States of America on acid-free paper
08 07 06 05   5 4 3
First Edition

Typeset in Palatino

American Psychiatric Publishing, Inc.
1000 Wilson Boulevard
Arlington, VA 22209-3901
www.appi.org

The correct citation for this book is
Ketter TA (editor): Advances in the Treatment of Bipolar Disorder (Review of Psychiatry Series, Volume 24, Number 3; Oldham JM and Riba MB, series editors). Washington, DC, American Psychiatric Publishing, 2005

Library of Congress Cataloging-in-Publication Data
Advances in treatment of bipolar disorder / edited by Terence A. Ketter. — 1st ed.
    p. ; cm. — (Review of psychiatry ; v. 24, no. 3)
  Includes bibliographical references and index.
  ISBN 1-58562-230-3 (pbk. : alk. paper)
1. Manic-depressive illness—Treatment
  [DNLM: 1. Bipolar Disorder—therapy.] I. Ketter, Terence A. II. Series: Review of psychiatry series ; v. 24, 3.

  RC516.A365 2004
  616.89'506—dc22

                                                        2005002205

British Library Cataloguing in Publication Data
A CIP record is available from the British Library.

Contents

Contributors

Julie Bonner, M.D.
Resident in Psychiatry, Department of Psychiatry and Behavioral Sciences, Stanford University School of Medicine, Stanford, California

Charles L. Bowden, M.D.
Professor of Psychiatry and Pharmacology, The University of Texas Health Science Center at San Antonio, San Antonio, Texas

Joseph R. Calabrese, M.D.
Professor of Psychiatry, Department of Psychiatry; Director, Mood Disorders Program, Case University School of Medicine, Cleveland, Ohio

Kiki D. Chang, M.D.
Assistant Professor of Psychiatry and Behavioral Sciences, Stanford University School of Medicine; Director, Pediatric Bipolar Disorders Research Program, Lucile Packard Children's Hospital, Stanford, California

Omar Elhaj, M.D.
Senior Research Fellow, Case University School of Medicine, University Hospitals of Cleveland, Cleveland, Ohio

Prashant Gajwani, M.D.
Assistant Professor of Psychiatry, Case University School of Medicine; Clinical Director, Mood Disorders Program, University Hospitals of Cleveland, Cleveland, Ohio

Keming Gao, M.D., Ph.D.
Bipolar Disorder Research Fellow, Case University School of Medicine, University Hospitals of Cleveland, Cleveland, Ohio

Meghan Howe, M.S.W.
Research Coordinator, Pediatric Bipolar Disorders Research Program, Stanford University, Stanford, California

Terence A. Ketter, M.D.
Professor of Psychiatry and Behavioral Sciences, Department of Psychiatry and Behavioral Sciences; Chief, Bipolar Disorders Clinic, Stanford University School of Medicine, Stanford, California

Wendy K. Marsh, M.D.
Research Fellow and Staff Physician, Department of Psychiatry and Behavioral Sciences, Stanford University School of Medicine, Stanford, California

David J. Muzina, M.D.
Director, Bipolar Disorders Clinical Research Program, Cleveland Clinic Foundation, Cleveland Clinic Lerner College of Medicine at Case University, Cleveland, Ohio

Cecylia Nowakowska, M.D., Ph.D.
Staff Psychiatrist, Department of Veterans Affairs, Palo Alto Healthcare System, Menlo Park, California

John M. Oldham, M.D., M.S.
Professor and Chair, Department of Psychiatry and Behavioral Sciences, Medical University of South Carolina, Charleston, South Carolina

Natalie L. Rasgon, M.D., Ph.D.
Associate Professor of Psychiatry and Obstetrics and Gynecology; Director, Behavioral Neuroendocrinology Program; Director, Women's Wellness Program, Department of Psychiatry and Behavioral Sciences, Stanford University School of Medicine, Stanford, California

Michelle B. Riba, M.D., M.S.
Clinical Professor and Associate Chair for Education and Academic Affairs, Department of Psychiatry, University of Michigan Medical School, Ann Arbor, Michigan

Gary S. Sachs, M.D.
Associate Professor of Psychiatry, Department of Psychiatry; Director, Bipolar Clinic and Research Program, Massachusetts General Hospital, Harvard Medical School, Boston, Massachusetts

Diana I. Simeonova, Dipl.-Psych.
Clinical Psychology Ph.D. Candidate, Department of Psychology, Emory University, Atlanta, Georgia

Vivek Singh, M.D.
Assistant Professor, The University of Texas Health Science Center at San Antonio, San Antonio, Texas

Po W. Wang, M.D.
Acting Assistant Professor of Psychiatry and Behavioral Sciences, Department of Psychiatry and Behavioral Sciences, Stanford University School of Medicine, Stanford, California

Laurel N. Zappert, B.A.
Clinical Research Associate, Behavioral Neuroendocrinology Program, Department of Psychiatry and Behavioral Sciences, Stanford University School of Medicine, Stanford, California

Introduction to the Review of Psychiatry Series

John M. Oldham, M.D., M.S.
Michelle B. Riba, M.D., M.S.

2005 REVIEW OF PSYCHIATRY SERIES TITLES

- *Psychiatric Genetics*
  EDITED BY KENNETH S. KENDLER, M.D., AND LINDON EAVES, PH.D., D.SC.
- *Sleep Disorders and Psychiatry*
  EDITED BY DANIEL J. BUYSSE, M.D.
- *Advances in Treatment of Bipolar Disorder*
  EDITED BY TERENCE A. KETTER, M.D.
- *Mood and Anxiety Disorders During Pregnancy and Postpartum*
  EDITED BY LEE S. COHEN, M.D., AND RUTA M. NONACS, M.D., PH.D.

The Annual Review of Psychiatry has been published for almost a quarter of a century, and 2005 marks the final year of publication of this highly successful series. First published in 1982, the Annual Review was conceived as a single volume highlighting new developments in the field that would be informative and of practical value to mental health practitioners. From the outset, the Annual Review was coordinated with the Annual Meeting of the American Psychiatric Association (APA), so that the material from each year's volume could also be presented in person by the chapter authors at the Annual Meeting. In its early years, the Review was one of a relatively small number of major books regularly published by American Psychiatric Press, Inc. (APPI; now American Psychiatric Publishing, Inc.). Through the subsequent years, however, the demand for new authoritative material led to an exponential growth in the number of new titles published by APPI each year. New published material became more readily available throughout each year, so that the unique function originally provided by the Annual Review was no longer needed.

Times change in many ways. The increased production volume, depth, and diversity of APPI's timely and authoritative material, now rapidly being augmented by electronic publishing, are welcome changes, and it is appropriate that this year's volume of the Annual Review represents the final curtain of the series. We have been privileged to be coeditors of the Annual Review for over a decade, and we are proud to have been a part of this distinguished series.

We hope you will agree that Volume 24 wonderfully lives up to the traditionally high standards of the Annual Review. In *Psychiatric Genetics*, edited by Kendler and Eaves, the fast-breaking and complex world of the genetics of psychiatric disorders is addressed. Following Kendler's clear and insightful introductory overview, Eaves, Chen, Neale, Maes, and Silberg present a careful analysis of the various methodologies used today to study the genetics of complex diseases in human populations. In turn, the book presents the latest findings on the genetics of schizophrenia, by Riley and Kendler; of anxiety disorders, by Hettema; of substance use disorders, by Prescott, Maes, and Kendler; and of antisocial behavior, by Jacobson.

Sleep Disorders and Psychiatry, edited by Buysse, brings us up to date on the sleep disorders from a psychiatric perspective, reviewing critically important clinical conditions that may not always receive the priority they deserve. Following a comprehensive introductory chapter, Buysse then presents, with his colleagues Germain, Moul, and Nofzinger, an authoritative review of the fundamental and pervasive problem of insomnia. Strollo and Davé next review sleep apnea, a potentially life-threatening condition that can also be an unrecognized source of excessive daytime sleepiness and impaired functioning. Black, Nishino, and Brooks present the basics of narcolepsy, along with new findings and treatment recommendations. In two separate chapters, Winkelman then reviews the parasomnias and the particular problem of restless legs syndrome. The book concludes with an extremely important chapter by Zee and Manthena reviewing circadian rhythm sleep disorders.

Advances in Treatment of Bipolar Disorder, edited by Ketter, provides an update on bipolar disorder. Following an introductory overview by Ketter, Sachs, Bowden, Calabrese, Chang, and Rasgon on the advances in the treatment of bipolar disorder, more specific material is presented on the treatment of acute mania, by Ketter, Wang, Nowakowska, Marsh, and Bonner. Sachs then presents a current look at the treatment of acute depression in bipolar patients, followed by a review by Bowden and Singh of the long-term management of bipolar disorder. The problem of rapid cycling is taken up by Muzina, Elhaj, Gajwani, Gao, and Calabrese. Chang, Howe, and Simeonova then discuss the treatment of children and adolescents with bipolar disorder, and the concluding chapter, by Rasgon and Zappert, provides a special focus on women with bipolar disorder.

Mood and Anxiety Disorders During Pregnancy and Postpartum, edited by Cohen and Nonacs, concerns the range of issues of psychiatric relevance related to pregnancy and the postpartum period. Cohen and Nonacs review the course of psychiatric illness during pregnancy, and the postpartum period is covered by Petrillo, Nonacs, Viguera, and Cohen. In this review, the authors focus particularly on depression, bipolar disorder, anxiety disorders, and psychotic disorders. The diagnosis and treatment of mood and anxiety disorders during pregnancy are then discussed in more detail in the subsequent chapter by Nonacs, Cohen, Viguera, and Mogielnicki, followed by a more in-depth look at management of bipolar disorder by Viguera, Cohen, Nonacs, and Baldessarini. Nonacs then presents a comprehensive and important look at the postpartum period, concentrating on mood disorders. This chapter is followed by a discussion of the use of antidepressants and mood-stabilizing medications during breast-feeding, by Ragan, Stowe, and Newport. Overall, this book provides up-to-date information about the management of common psychiatric disorders during gestation and during the critical postpartum period.

Before closing this final version of our annual introductory comments, we would like to thank all of the authors who have contributed so generously to the Annual Review, as well as the editors who preceded us. In addition, we thank the wonderful staff at APPI who have so diligently helped produce a quality product each year, and we would particularly like to thank our two administrative assistants, Liz Bednarowicz and Linda Gacioch, without whom the work could not have been done.

Chapter 1

Introduction

Terence A. Ketter, M.D.
Gary S. Sachs, M.D.
Charles L. Bowden, M.D.
Joseph R. Calabrese, M.D.
Kiki D. Chang, M.D.
Natalie L. Rasgon, M.D., Ph.D.

An increasing number of therapies are becoming available for patients with bipolar disorders. Lithium was reported to be effective in acute mania in 1949, and saw widespread use in Europe by the 1960s, but was only approved for the treatment of acute mania by the U.S. Food and Drug Administration (FDA) in 1970. Chlorpromazine was approved by the FDA for the treatment of acute mania in the United States in 1973, and the next year, lithium received a maintenance indication for the treatment of patients with bipolar disorders. The anticonvulsants carbamazepine and valproate were increasingly used off-label for bipolar disorders in the 1980s and 1990s, respectively. The divalproex formulation of the latter was approved by the FDA for the treatment of acute mania in the United States in 1994. Since 2000 there has been rapid further evolution of the field, with multiple potential new medications and adjunctive psychosocial interventions being assessed for utility in the treatment of bipolar disorders.

Table 1–1 lists treatments for bipolar disorders approved by the FDA for use in adults. As such approval generally requires at least two adequately sized, multicenter, randomized, double-blind, placebo-controlled trials demonstrating efficacy and safety, these medications are typically considered the most well-established

Table 1–1. Agents approved for bipolar disorder in the United States

Acute mania		Maintenance		Acute depression	
Year	Drug	Year	Drug	Year	Drug
1970	Lithium	1974	Lithium	2003	Olanzapine-
1973	Chlorpromazine	2003	Lamotrigine		fluoxetine
1994	Divalproex	2004	Olanzapine		combination
2000	Olanzapine*	2005	Aripiprazole		
2003	Risperidone*				
2004	Quetiapine*				
2004	Ziprasidone				
2004	Aripiprazole				
2004	Carbamazepine				

*Adjunctive as well as monotherapy

management options. However, due to the amount of time required to obtain FDA indications, this list may not include treatment options that already have comparable (two adequately sized, multicenter, randomized, double-blind, placebo-controlled trials) or emerging (one adequately sized, multicenter, randomized, double-blind, placebo-controlled trial) substantial evidence of efficacy and tolerability.

Examination of Table 1–1 reveals that although there are multiple treatments (nine) indicated for acute mania, there are only a few (four) approved for maintenance therapy, and only one indicated for acute bipolar depression. Thus, although the field is rapidly advancing (over two-thirds of the 14 indications have been obtained since 2000), there still remain important limitations in the number of approved treatment options for acute bipolar depression, maintenance treatment, and the diverse combinations of medications commonly encountered in clinical practice.

Hence, clinical needs commonly exceed the management options supported by FDA indications. In such instances, the next best-established treatments are those supported by at least one adequately sized, randomized, controlled trial. Table 1–2 provides a schema regarding the quality of evidence supporting the

Table 1–2. Controlled acute mania and depression studies[a]

	Effective[a]	Inadequate data	No controlled data	Ineffective
Acute mania	Aripiprazole Carbamazepine Chlorpromazine Divalproex Haloperidol Lithium Olanzapine Quetiapine Risperidone Ziprasidone	ECT Oxcarbazepine Phenytoin	Clozapine Levetiracetam Tiagabine[b] Zonisamide	Gabapentin Lamotrigine Topiramate
Acute depression	Lamotrigine Lithium Olanzapine (modest) Olanzapine + fluoxetine Quetiapine	Antidepressants[c] Carbamazepine Divalproex ECT Gabapentin Mifepristone Pramipexole T_3, T_4	Aripiprazole Chlorpromazine Clozapine Haloperidol Levetiracetam Oxcarbazepine Penytoin Risperidone	

Table 1–2. Controlled acute mania and depression studies[a] *(continued)*

	Effective[a]	Inadequate data	No controlled data	Ineffective
Acute depression *(continued)*		Topiramate Tranylcypromine	Tiagabine Ziprasidone Zonisamide	

[a] Active treatment $N > 40$
[b] Negative small open trial
[c] Adjunctive, other than olanzapine plus fluoxetine combinatin

use of various medications for acute mania and acute bipolar depression in adults. In this schema, treatments that have evidence from at least one adequately sized (at least 40 patients receiving the active treatment considered), multicenter, randomized, double-blind, placebo-controlled trial are considered "effective" (if positive) or "ineffective" (if negative). Medications with less compelling (most often due to sample size limitations) controlled data are described as having "inadequate data," and treatments with "no controlled data" are also listed.

Examination of Table 1–2 reveals that although there are multiple treatments (ten) with adequate controlled data supporting efficacy for acute mania, there are only a few (five) with such data indicating efficacy for acute bipolar depression. Importantly, many treatments have either inadequate or no controlled data, particularly with respect to efficacy in acute bipolar depression.

There are two main categories of new potential medication treatment options for bipolar disorders, namely, newer antipsychotics and anticonvulsants. Newer antipsychotics generally appear effective for acute mania, and emerging data suggest potential utility for these agents in maintenance treatment and acute bipolar depression (Table 1–3). In contrast, newer anticonvulsants appear to have diverse psychotropic profiles, and although (with the possible exception of oxcarbazepine) not generally effective for acute mania, these agents may have utility for other aspects of bipolar disorders or comorbid conditions (Table 1–4).

Advances in the treatment of bipolar disorders have been sufficiently rapid that even relatively recent efforts to summarize management options for clinicians, such as the 2002 revision of the *American Psychiatric Association Practice Guideline for the Treatment of Patients With Bipolar Disorder*, quickly become outdated. In this volume we review recent developments, emphasizing interventions supported by controlled studies.

Chapter 2, by Ketter and associates, describes these substantial recent advances in the treatment of acute mania. Since 2000, five newer antipsychotics (olanzapine, risperidone, quetiapine, ziprasidone, and aipiprazole) received monotherapy, and three (olanzapine, risperidone, and quetiapine) received adjunctive

Table 1–3. Emerging roles of newer antipsychotics in patients with bipolar disorders

As primary therapies for bipolar disorders
- Olanzapine: mania, maintenance, depression (combined with fluoxetine)
- Risperidone: mania
- Quetiapine: mania, ± depression
- Ziprasidone: mania
- Aripiprazole: mania, ± maintenance

As adjuncts for bipolar disorders
- Olanzapine: mania
- Risperidone: mania
- Quetiapine: mania
- Clozapine: treatment resistant

Table 1–4. Emerging diverse roles of anticonvulsants in patients with bipolar disorders

As primary therapies for bipolar disorders
- Divalproex: mania, ± maintenance, ± rapid cycling
- Carbamazepine: mania, ± maintenance, ± rapid cycling
- Lamotrigine: maintenance, ± depression, ± rapid cycling
- Oxcarbazepine: ± mania

As adjuncts for comorbid conditions
- Benzodiazepines: anxiety, insomnia, agitation
- Gabapentin: anxiety, insomnia, pain
- Topiramate: obesity, eating disorders, migraine, alcoholism
- Zonisamide: ± obesity, ± eating disorders

(added to lithium or divalproex) indications for acute mania. Also, in late 2004, a proprietary beaded, extended-release capsule formulation of carbamazepine received a monotherapy indication for acute mania. Lithium, divalproex, and carbamazepine remain important treatment options for acute mania. Controlled trials to date suggest that newer anticonvulsants (with the possible exception of oxcarbazepine) are not generally effective for acute mania, but may have utility for other aspects of bipolar disorders (such as lamotrigine for maintenance treatment or acute bipolar depression), or comorbid conditions (such as gabapentin for anxiety or pain; topiramate for obesity, eating disorders, migraine prevention, and alcohol dependence; and zonisamide for obesity).

Sachs considers recent developments in the treatment of acute bipolar depression in Chapter 3. Therapeutic options beyond mood stabilizers are needed as lithium, divalproex, and carbamazepine efficacy in acute bipolar depression appears more modest than in acute mania. The first treatment for this indication (olanzapine plus fluoxetine combination) received FDA approval in 2003. Emerging data suggest efficacy for lamotrigine and quetiapine for acute bipolar depression, and it is anticipated that adequate controlled trials for additional agents will occur in the near future. Although adjunctive antidepressants are commonly used in acute bipolar depression, the evidence supporting this practice is less compelling, and more research is clearly needed.

Chapter 4, by Bowden and Singh, explores recent advances in the maintenance treatment of patients with bipolar disorder. Lithium and divalproex remain important treatment options. In 2003 lamotrigine became the first new treatment in 29 years to receive FDA approval for this indication, the following year olanzapine was also approved, and in early 2005 aripiprazole was approved. It is anticipated that adequate controlled trials for additional medications will occur in the near future. Moreover, emerging controlled data suggest the efficacy of adjunctive psychosocial therapies as maintenance treatments for bipolar disorder. Long-term treatment compared to acute treatment provides distinctive opportunities and challenges with respect to managing the adverse effects of medication, and maintaining the therapeutic alliance, treatment adherence, and involvement of significant others to enhance outcomes.

In Chapter 5, Muzina and associates describe recent developments in the treatment of patients with rapid-cycling bipolar disorder. To date, no treatment has received FDA approval for patients with this subtype of bipolar disorder, however, results of controlled trials are beginning to provide clinically relevant insights into the management of patients with rapid cycling. Although older data suggested that divalproex and carbamazepine may be more effective than lithium in bipolar disorder patients with rapid cycling, emerging data indicate that this illness subtype may be generally resistant to such treatments, even when combinations of medications are used. Controlled data support the efficacy of lamotrigine among bipolar II patients with rapid cycling, and more limited evidence suggests that the potential efficacy of atypical antipsychotics such as olanzapine and quetiapine in patients with rapid cycling is worth systematically exploring.

Chapter 6, by Chang and associates, describes recent advances in the treatment of children and adolescents with bipolar disorder. To date, no treatment has received FDA approval for this challenging subgroup of patients with bipolar disorder, and controlled data are limited. Nevertheless, recent research is yielding information with important management implications, regarding the utility of mood stabilizers, atypical antipsychotics, adjunctive psychotherapy, and combination treatments in children and adolescents with bipolar disorder. Therapeutic challenges include devising optimal interventions to manage comorbid disruptive behavior disorders, anxiety disorders, and substance use disorders, and perhaps in the future to prevent the development of syndromal illness in individuals at risk, such as offspring of parents with bipolar disorders.

The final chapter, by Rasgon and Zappert, describes recent advances in the treatment of bipolar disorder in women, a subgroup of patients who historically have been inadequately studied. Controlled data in this area remain limited, but recent research has yielded information with substantive clinical implications. Thus, important gender differences in the phenomenology and management of bipolar disorders in women compared to men are beginning to be understood, and emerging data are starting to clarify relationships between the menstrual cycle and mood disturbance that can significantly impact illness course. Specific treatment considerations for women with bipolar disorder include pharmacological management of bipolar disorder during pregnancy and postpartum, management of medication induced effects on reproductive function, as well as evaluation of mood effects of hormonal contraceptives.

Recent research not only has helped us better understand the utility of older medications but also has provided clinicians with important new treatment options for bipolar disorders. Efforts to provide evidence-based care have been substantively facilitated by data from the recent controlled trials described in this volume. Although progress has been encouraging, clinical needs continue to exceed the treatment options supported by controlled data, and additional research is required to allow further progress in addressing the challenges facing clinicians caring for patients with bipolar disorders.

Chapter 2

Treatment of Acute Mania in Bipolar Disorder

Terence A. Ketter, M.D.
Po W. Wang, M.D.
Cecylia Nowakowska, M.D., Ph.D.
Wendy K. Marsh, M.D.
Julie Bonner, M.D.

Treatment options for patients with acute mania are evolving at an accelerating rate. Over a period of 24 years, the U.S. Food and Drug Administration (FDA) approved the first three agents for monotherapy treatment of acute mania (lithium in 1970, chlorpromazine in 1973, and divalproex in 1994). Between 2000 and 2004, five newer antipsychotics (olanzapine, risperidone, quetiapine, ziprasidone, and aripiprazole) received monotherapy indications and three (olanzapine, risperidone, and quetiapine) received adjunctive indications for acute mania, based on multiple multicenter, randomized, double-blind, placebo-controlled and active-comparator-controlled clinical trials (Figures 2–1 and 2–2). Also, in late 2004, a proprietary beaded, extended-release capsule formulation of carbamazepine received a monotherapy indication for acute mania. In addition, there have been multiple controlled trials of anticonvulsants in acute mania; however, to date, only divalproex and carbamazepine and possibly oxcarbazepine appear effective.

In this chapter, we review the research on pharmacological treatment of mania, focusing on recent controlled studies. In addition to lithium, divalproex, and carbamazepine, we consider two potential new treatment categories for acute mania: newer

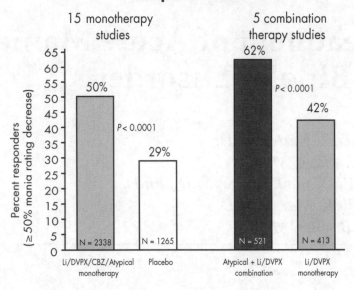

Figure 2–1. Overview of 20 acute mania studies.

Pooled data from 15 recent monotherapy (*left*, see Figure 2–2 caption for citations) and 5 recent combination (newer antipsychotic plus lithium/divalproex) (Sachs et al. 2002; Tohen et al. 2002b; Yatham et al. 2003, in press) therapy (*right*) acute mania studies. Monotherapy yielded an approximately 20% increase in pooled response rate compared with placebo (combined with acute hospitalization and a few days of rescue benzodiazepine) (50% versus 29%). Combination therapy yielded an approximately 20% increase in pooled response rate compared with monotherapy (62% versus 42%).

Note. Li=lithium, DVPX=divalproex, CBZ=carbamazepine.

antipsychotics and newer anticonvulsants. Such research is helping to refine our knowledge regarding lithium, divalproex, and carbamazepine, enhancing our appreciation the utility of newer antipsychotics, and helping us understand the limitations of newer anticonvulsants in acute mania. Newer antipsychotics generally appear effective for acute mania (Figures 2–1 and 2–2), whereas anticonvulsants appear to have diverse psychotropic profiles, and although not effective for acute mania (with the possible exception of oxcarbazepine), they may have utility for other aspects of bipolar disorders or comorbid conditions.

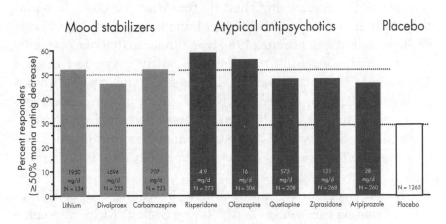

Figure 2–2. Overview of 15 acute mania monotherapy studies.
Pooled data from recent controlled trials of the mood stabilizers lithium
(Bowden et al. 1994; Bowden et al., in review), divalproex (Bowden et al. 1994;
Tohen et al. 2002a; Zajecka et al. 2002), and carbamazepine (Weisler et al. 2004b;
Weisler et al., in review), and the newer antipsychotics olanzapine (Tohen et al.
1999, 2000, 2002a; Zajecka et al. 2002), risperidone (Hirschfeld et al. 2003a; Khan-
na et al. 2003), quetiapine (Calabrese et al., in review), ziprasidone (Potkin et al.
2004), and aripiprazole (Keck et al. 2003a; Sachs et al. 2004b), as well as placebo
(Bowden et al. 1994, in review; Calabrese et al., in review; Hirschfeld et al. 2003b;
Keck et al. 2003a; Khanna et al. 2003; Potkin et al. 2004; Sachs et al. 2004b; Tohen
et al. 1999, 2000; Weisler et al. 2004b, in review). Active treatments had response
(greater than 50% mania rating decrease) rates of about 50%, whereas placebo
yielded a pooled response rate of about 30%.

Lithium

Lithium received FDA approval for the treatment of manic episodes of manic-depressive illness in 1970. Early studies of lithium
in acute mania had randomized (Maggs 1963; Schou et al. 1954)
and nonrandomized (Goodwin et al. 1969; Stokes et al. 1971)
crossover designs, yet despite these methodological differences
and limitations, they consistently found that about 80% of patients with acute mania responded to lithium. Subsequent multicenter, randomized, double-blind, placebo-controlled trials of
other medications using lithium as an active-comparator have
confirmed lithium to be effective in acute mania, albeit at times

with somewhat lower response rates than in earlier studies. In one 3-week acute mania study (Bowden et al. 1994), the response (at least 50% decrease in Schedule for Affective Disorders and Schizophrenia–Change [SADS-C] Mania Rating Scale score) rate of 36 patients given lithium (49%) was similar to that of 69 patients given divalproex (48%) and significantly exceeded that of 74 patients given placebo (25%). In this study, mean peak lithium dosage was 1,950 mg/day, mean final serum lithium concentration was 1.2 mEq/L, and lithium adverse effects included vomiting and twitching, with 11% of participants discontinuing because of adverse effects (versus 6% with divalproex and 3% with placebo).

In a 12-week acute mania study (Bowden et al. 2005), response rate on the Young Mania Rating Scale (YMRS) at week 3 for 98 patients given lithium (53%) was similar to that of the 107 patients given quetiapine (53%) and significantly exceeded that of 95 patients given placebo (27%). At week 12, lithium (76%) and quetiapine (72%) response rates still exceeded that of placebo (41%). In this study, the mean final serum lithium concentration was 0.77 mEq/L. Lithium therapy was associated with tremor, insomnia, and headache, with 6.1% discontinuing due to adverse events versus 6.5% with quetiapine and 4.1% with placebo.

In a failed 3-week acute mania study in which antipsychotics were allowed for the first 5 days (Bowden et al. 2000), SADS-C Mania Rating Scale response rates were similar among the 36 patients given lithium (42%), the 95 patients given placebo (46%), and the 85 patients given low-dose (final dosage 50 mg/day) lamotrigine (44%). However, in a 6-week add-on study in which antipsychotics were allowed up to week 3, the response rate for 77 patients given lithium (62%) was significantly higher than for the 77 patients given placebo (47%), whereas the response rate of 74 patients given lamotrigine (final dosage 200 mg/day; 55%) failed to achieve statistical separation from placebo (Bowden et al. 2000). In these studies, lithium serum concentrations ranged between 0.8 and 1.3 mEq/L.

In 2003 and 2004, three newer antipsychotics (olanzapine, risperidone, and quetiapine) were approved for use in combination with lithium (or divalproex) for treatment of acute mania. Randomized, double-blind, placebo-controlled acute mania studies have indicated efficacy when olanzapine (Tohen et al. 2002b), risperidone (Sachs et al. 2002; Yatham et al. 2003), or quetiapine (Sachs et al. 2004a; Yatham et al. 2004) are added to lithium (or divalproex). In these studies serum lithium concentrations ranged between 0.7 and 0.82 mEq/L, and the addition of a newer antipsychotic tended to yield slightly more adverse effects. In response to these studies, the American Psychiatric Association (2002) revised its practice guideline for treatment of bipolar disorder, adding recommendations for combined use of antipsychotics and mood stabilizers as first-line interventions in severe acute mania.

To limit early adverse effects, lithium for acute mania is commonly introduced at lower (600–900 mg/day) dosages and gradually increased until therapeutic efficacy is adequate, adverse effects supervene, or serum concentrations exceed 1.2 mEq/L. Euthymic or depressed patients, compared with manic patients, tend to be less able to tolerate adverse effects and thus may require even more gradual initiation. Response to lithium in acute mania tends to occur with serum concentrations between 0.8 and 1.2 mEq/L.

Lithium limitations include common adverse effects, such as tremor, polyuria, and polydipsia, that can occur within the range of therapeutic serum concentrations (0.8–1.2 mEq/L). Increasingly problematic diarrhea, vomiting, drowsiness, muscular weakness, and impaired coordination can occur with higher levels, and severe adverse effects involving multiple organ systems emerge at concentrations greater than 2.0 mEq/L. Lithium dosages of less than 1,000 mg/day are usually well tolerated, whereas dosages above 2,000 mg/day commonly yield side effects, but adverse effects are more closely related to lithium serum concentrations than to dosage. Thus the product information for lithium in the United States includes a "black-box" warning that lithium toxicity is closely related to serum lithium concentrations and can occur at dosages close to therapeutic levels. The product information also includes a warning to avoid lithium in patients with significant renal or cardiovascular disease, severe debilitation or dehydration, or sodium depletion, because the risk of lithium toxicity is very high. Other warnings include the risk of adverse renal effects, including nephrogenic diabetes insipidus, glomerular and interstitial fibrosis with chronic lithium therapy, and cases of encephalopathy with combinations of lithium and neuroleptics.

Extended-release—compared with immediate-release—lithium formulations may attenuate adverse effects in general by yielding lower peak serum concentrations and may reduce upper gastrointestinal adverse effects (nausea and vomiting) by delaying absorption. However, extended-release formulations can exacerbate lower gastrointestinal problems (such as diarrhea) because of the delay in absorption. Laboratory monitoring of serum lithium concentrations as well as thyroid and renal function is necessary because thyroid and renal adverse effects can also occur. As discussed in Chapter 7, lithium is also teratogenic (FDA Pregnancy Category D due to cardiac malformations in about 1%).

Physiological conditions, medical disorders, and drug interactions can increase serum lithium concentrations, potentially yielding toxicity. Serum lithium concentrations may rise with dehydration, sodium depletion, advanced age, renal disease, and concomitant administration of angiotensin-converting enzyme inhibitors, metronidazole, thiazide diuretics, and nonsteroidal anti-inflammatory drugs.

Divalproex

Divalproex received FDA approval for the treatment of manic episodes associated with bipolar disorder in 1994. An early, small, single-center, randomized, double-blind, placebo-controlled trial found divalproex effective in acute mania in patients with a history of lithium resistance (Pope et al. 1991). In this study, 17 patients given valproate had a YMRS response rate (53%) significantly higher than that of 19 patients given placebo (11%). Divalproex adverse effects included nausea, vomiting, and sedation, with 12% discontinuing due to adverse events (versus 5.3% with placebo).

A larger multicenter, randomized, double-blind, placebo-controlled, acute mania trial (Bowden et al. 1994) found divalproex effective, with 69 patients given divalproex having a SAD-C Mania Rating Scale response rate (48%) similar to that of 36 patients given lithium (49%) and significantly exceeding that of 74 patients given placebo (25%). In this study, 42% of patients had histories of lithium failure. Mean peak divalproex dosage was about 2,000 mg/day. Mean final serum valproate concentration was 93 μg/mL. Divalproex adverse effects included vomiting, with 6% discontinuing due to adverse effects (versus 11% with lithium and 3% with placebo). Serum valproate concentrations between 45 and 100 μg/mL were associated with antimanic response, with some patients able to tolerate and obtain additional benefit with concentrations up to 125 μg/mL (Bowden et al. 1996).

In a small, single-center, randomized, double-blind, active-comparator trial (Freeman et al. 1992), lithium and valproate both appeared to relieve manic symptoms, but lithium was slightly more efficacious, with 13 patients given lithium having a SAD-C Mania Rating Scale response rate (92%) higher than that of 14 patients given valproate (64%). In patients given lithium (but not valproate), mixed episodes were associated with less favorable responses. Final serum lithium concentrations ranged between 0.8 and 1.4 mEq/L, whereas mean final serum valproate concentration was 98 μg/mL.

Thus divalproex appears to have a broader spectrum of efficacy than lithium, yielding benefit in patients with histories of lithium failure (Bowden et al. 1994; Pope et al. 1991) and lithium-resistant illness, such as patients with dysphoric manic (Freeman et al. 1992; Swann et al. 1997) or mixed (Bowden et al. 1994) episodes and those with multiple prior episodes (Swann et al. 2000).

Two multicenter, randomized, double-blind, active-comparator studies suggested that there was a modest tolerability (less sedation and weight gain) advantage for divalproex compared with olanzapine and a slight efficacy advantage for olanzapine in acute mania (Tohen et al. 2002a; Zajecka et al. 2002). One of these reports (Tohen et al. 2002a) described a 3-week study in which the YMRS response rate was lower in 126 patients given divalproex (42%) than in 125 patients given olanzapine (54%). Olanzapine was started at 15 mg/day with a mean final dosage of 17 mg/

day, and divalproex was gradually introduced at 750 mg/day with a mean final dosage of 1,401 mg/day. Mean final serum valproate concentration was 84 µg/mL. Divalproex yielded less somnolence, dry mouth, increased appetite, tremor, slurred speech, and mean weight increase (0.9 versus 2.5 kg) and fewer discontinuations for adverse events (7.1% versus 9.6%) than olanzapine, but divalproex produced more nausea.

Another report (Zajecka et al. 2002) described a 12-week study in which the SAD-C Mania Rating Scale response rate was lower in 60 patients given divalproex (53%) than in 55 patients given olanzapine (62%). Olanzapine was started at 10 mg/day with a mean final dosage of 15 mg/day, and divalproex was rapidly introduced (starting at 20 mg/kg/day), yielding mean serum valproate concentrations of 78, 97, and 101 µg/mL on days 3, 6, and 10, respectively. Mean final divalproex dosage was 1,956 mg/day, yielding a mean final serum valproate concentration of 78 µg/mL. Divalproex yielded less somnolence, weight gain, rhinitis, edema, slurred speech, and mean weight increase (2.5 versus 4.0 kg) than olanzapine but had more discontinuations for adverse events (11% versus 9%), although no adverse events were reported in a significantly greater proportion of divalproex-treated compared with olanzapine-treated subjects.

In 2003 and 2004, olanzapine, risperidone, and quetiapine were approved for use in combination with divalproex (or lithium) for acute mania. Randomized, double-blind, placebo-controlled acute mania studies have indicated efficacy when olanzapine (Tohen et al. 2002b), risperidone (Sachs et al. 2002; Yatham et al. 2003), and quetiapine (Delbello et al. 2002; Sachs et al. 2004b; Yatham et al., in press) were added to divalproex (or lithium). In these studies serum valproate concentrations ranged between 64 and 104 µg/mL, and the addition of a newer antipsychotic tended to yield somewhat more adverse effects.

In one multicenter, randomized, double-blind, placebo-controlled, 3-week acute mania study (Muller-Oerlinghausen et al. 2000), the YMRS response rate for 69 patients given valproate (mean dosage 20 mg/kg/day, mean serum concentration 80 µg/mL) combined with antipsychotics (primarily haloperidol and/or perazine) was 70%, significantly higher than the 46% response rate of the 67 patients given placebo plus antipsychotics. In this study, co-therapy with valproate was associated with lower antipsychotic dosages and was generally well tolerated, with asthenia the only adverse effect more common with combination therapy and a low rate of discontinuation for adverse events (2.9% versus 3.0% with monotherapy).

As mentioned earlier, the APA practice guideline now recommends combinations of antipsychotics and mood stabilizers as first-line interventions for the treatment of severe cases of acute mania (American Psychiatric Association 2002). Recent studies are helping to further refine our knowledge of the clinical utility of divalproex in bipolar disorders. For instance, divalproex oral loading (initiating at 20–30 mg/kg/day for 2 days and then 20 mg/kg/day) rapidly yielded therapeutic (50–125 µg/mL) blood concentrations and appeared to be rapidly effective and well tolerated in acute mania (Hirschfeld et al. 2003a). This approach has the potential to more expediently address symptoms of acute mania than the less-aggressive approach (starting at 750 mg/day in divided doses) described in the product information.

Divalproex tends to be somewhat better tolerated than lithium or carbamazepine, with central nervous system and gastrointestinal problems being the most common adverse effects. Recent studies and post-marketing experience are refining our appreciation of the tolerability limitations of divalproex. Specifically, the product information in the United States has been revised to add rare pancreatitis to the black-box warnings of teratogenicity (FDA Pregnancy Category D due to spina bifida in about 1–2%) and rare hepatoxicity. As noted in Chapter 7, recent data suggest that rates of malformations with divalproex could be higher compared to rates with lamotrigine or compared to rates with no anticonvulsant exposure (Alsdorf et al. 2004; Cunnington 2004; Vajda et al. 2004). Other warnings in the product information include the risks of hyperammonemic encephalopathy in patients with rare urea cycle disorders, increased somnolence in the elderly, and thrombocytopenia. In the United States, an extended-release divalproex formulation was approved in 2000 for the prevention of migraine headaches (but not to date for acute mania). This formulation has the potential to yield fewer adverse effects (such as gastrointestinal disturbance or tremor), allowing less frequent dosing and thus better adherence.

There have been varying reports for more than a decade regarding a possible association between valproate therapy and polycystic ovarian syndrome (PCOS) in women with epilepsy (Isojarvi et al. 1993; Rasgon 2004). Two recent studies of patients with bipolar disorder showed a modest (8%–10%) risk of PCOS in women with bipolar disorder (Altshuler et al. 2004; Joffe et al. 2004), indicating a need for prospective trials to systematically assess this issue (see Chapter 7).

Valproate has some drug–drug interactions, as it can inhibit metabolism of other drugs, including lamotrigine and the active carbamazepine epoxide metabolite. Moreover, valproate is susceptible to enzyme inducers; thus, carbamazepine decreases valproate serum concentrations.

Carbamazepine

In contrast to valproate, multicenter, randomized, double-blind, placebo-controlled trials have only recently confirmed the efficacy of a proprietary beaded, extended-release capsule formulation of carbamazepine (ERC-CBZ) in acute mania (Weisler et al. 2004a, in press). One of these (Weisler et al. 2004a) was a 3-week study in which the YMRS response rate was greater in 101 patients given ERC-CBZ (42%) than in 103 patients given placebo (22%). ERC-CBZ yielded a significantly greater mean YMRS decrease by day 14. ERC-CBZ was started at 200 mg twice a day and titrated by daily increments of 200 mg, with a mean final ERC-CBZ dosage of 756 mg/day and a mean final serum carbamazepine concentration of 8.9 μg/mL. Discontinuation for adverse events was noted in 12.9% of patients given ERC-CBZ and 5.8% of patients given placebo. The other study (Weisler et al., in press) had the same design, and the YMRS response rate was greater in 122 patients given ERC-CBZ (61%) than in 117 patients given placebo (29%). ERC-CBZ yielded a significantly greater mean YMRS decrease by day 7; mean final dosage of ERC-CBZ was 666 mg/day. Discontinuation for adverse events was noted in 9.0% of those given ERC-CBZ and 5.1% of those given placebo. For both studies, ERC-CBZ adverse effects included dizziness, nausea, and somnolence.

These studies resulted in an FDA monotherapy indication for ERC-CBZ for the treatment of acute mania in late 2004. However, the absence of an FDA indication prior to late 2004 and its complexity of use have thus far led carbamazepine to be considered an alternative rather than a first-line intervention in bipolar disorders (American Psychiatric Association 2002).

Older studies suggested utility for carbamazepine combined with lithium (Kramlinger and Post 1989) or antipsychotics (Okuma et al. 1989) in the treatment of acute mania. However, carbamazepine can increase the hepatic metabolism of multiple other agents, potentially compromising the efficacy of combination therapies (Ketter et al. 1991a, 1991b). In a recent study that reemphasized this point, carbamazepine yielded substantial decreases in blood risperidone concentrations, compromising the efficacy of the combination for treatment of acute mania (Yatham et al. 2003).

To limit early adverse effects, carbamazepine is commonly introduced at low (100–400 mg/day) dosages and gradually increased until therapeutic efficacy is adequate, adverse effects supervene, or serum concentrations exceed 12 μg/mL. Euthymic or depressed patients tend to be less able than manic patients to tolerate adverse effects and thus may require more gradual initiation. Although response in bipolar disorder does not appear related to serum concentrations, the 4–12 μg/mL range used in epilepsy may be considered a broad target, and serum carbamazepine concentrations may be used as pharmacokinetic checks for extreme values.

Carbamazepine has several important limitations and has a black-box warning in its product information regarding the risks of rare aplastic anemia and agranulocytosis. Carbamazepine is also associated with common benign leukopenia, which in rare instances may be an early indication of serious blood dyscrasia. Other warnings in the product information include the risks of teratogenicity, rare serious rashes, and increased intraocular pressure due to mild anticholinergic activity. As discussed in

Chapter 7, carbamazepine has the potential for teratogenicity (FDA Pregnancy Category D due to craniofacial defects, fingernail hypoplasia, and developmental delay in about 11%–26% and spina bifida in about 3%). Carbamazepine is also associated with common benign rashes, which in rare instances may be harbingers of rare, more serious rashes. However, in occasional patients carbamazepine may be better tolerated than other agents, and data continue to support the notion that one potential advantage of carbamazepine is the low risk of clinically significant weight gain (Ketter et al. 2004).

Carbamazepine drug–drug interactions can yield carbamazepine toxicity (e.g., when erythromycin or valproate is added to carbamazepine) and reduce the efficacy of other medications (e.g., hormonal contraceptives and multiple psychotropic drugs, including several newer anticonvulsants and newer antipsychotics) (Ketter et al. 1991a, 1991b).

Newer Antipsychotics

Between 2000 and 2004, five newer antipsychotics (olanzapine, risperidone, quetiapine, ziprasidone, and aripiprazole) received FDA monotherapy indications for acute mania. Moreover, as mentioned previously, in 2003 and 2004, olanzapine, risperidone, and quetiapine also received FDA adjunctive therapy indications for acute mania.

Clozapine

Although clozapine lacks an FDA indication for acute mania, this medication is of interest not only because it is the prototypical atypical antipsychotic but also because it is the only agent approved for treatment-resistant schizophrenia and for decreasing suicidal behavior in patients with schizophrenia (Meltzer et al. 2003).

Uncontrolled reports (for a review see Frye et al. 1998) and one controlled trial (Suppes et al. 1999) suggested that clozapine may have efficacy in bipolar disorders. In a 1-year randomized open trial, clozapine plus treatment as usual was superior to treatment as usual without clozapine in patients with treatment-resistant bipolar I and schizoaffective disorder, bipolar type (Suppes et al. 1999). Mean clozapine dosage was lower in bipolar I (234 mg/day) than in schizoaffective disorder, bipolar type (623 mg/day) patients, and only 3 of 19 (16%) clozapine patients discontinued due to adverse effects.

However, clozapine has a challenging adverse effect profile compared with other treatment options. The product information includes black-box warnings regarding the risks of agranulocytosis, seizures, myocarditis, and other cardiovascular and respiratory adverse effects. Thus, this agent tends to be held in reserve for patients with treatment-resistant bipolar disorders. Increasing concerns have been raised regarding the risks of hyperglycemia and diabetes mellitus with clozapine and newer antipsychotics. Indeed, the FDA has stipulated changes in the product information not only for clozapine but also for olanzapine, risperidone, quetiapine, ziprasidone, and aripiprazole to reflect these risks, which suggests a class effect for such problems. In contrast, the report of a recent consensus development conference on antipsychotics and obesity, diabetes, and hyperlipidemia emphasized differences between agents, with clozapine and olanzapine being the most implicated, followed by risperidone and quetiapine, and with ziprasidone and aripiprazole being the least implicated (American Diabetes Association et al. 2004). Thus, clinical and (as indicated) laboratory monitoring for obesity, diabetes, and hyperlipidemia appears prudent for patients receiving clozapine. Other warnings in the product information include the risks of eosinophilia and neuroleptic malignant syndrome. To date, clozapine has not been associated with congenital malformations in humans (FDA Pregnancy Category B).

Clozapine has some drug–drug interactions, as certain enzyme inducers such as carbamazepine can decrease, and some enzyme inhibitors such as macrolide antibiotics may increase, serum clozapine concentrations. In addition, combining clozapine with bone marrow suppressants is not recommended due to concerns regarding the potential for increasing the risk of agranulocytosis.

Olanzapine

Olanzapine received FDA approval for monotherapy treatment of acute manic or mixed episodes associated with bipolar disorder in 2000 and for short-term combination therapy (with lithium or valproate) in 2003. Emerging data suggest that olanzapine may have utility in other phases of bipolar disorders. As noted in Chapter 4, olanzapine received an indication for maintenance monotherapy for bipolar disorder in 2004. Also, as described in Chapter 3 by Sachs, in late 2003, the combination of olanzapine with fluoxetine became the first treatment approved for acute bipolar depression.

Substantial evidence supports the efficacy of olanzapine in acute mania. Multicenter, randomized, double-blind, placebo-controlled trials indicate that olanzapine is effective in acute mania both as monotherapy (Tohen et al. 1999, 2000) and as adjunctive treatment (added to lithium or valproate) (Tohen et al. 2002b). The first monotherapy acute mania study (Tohen et al. 1999) was a 3-week trial in which the YMRS response rate was greater in 69 patients given olanzapine (49%) than in 70 patients given placebo (24%). Olanzapine was started at 10 mg/day, and the mean modal dosage was 15 mg/day. Olanzapine yielded a significantly greater mean YMRS decrease by day 21 compared with placebo. Olanzapine adverse effects included somnolence, dry mouth, dizziness, and weight gain (+1.65 kg with olanzapine versus −0.44 kg with placebo), but no patients discontinued olanzapine due to adverse events (versus 2.9% with placebo).

The second acute mania monotherapy study (Tohen et al. 2000) lasted 4 weeks, and the YMRS response rate was greater in 55 patients given olanzapine (65%) than in 60 patients given placebo (43%). Olanzapine was started at 15 mg/day, and the mean modal dosage was 16 mg/day. Starting at a higher dosage than in the first study appeared to accelerate the onset of efficacy, because olanzapine yielded a significantly greater mean YMRS decrease by day 7 compared with placebo in this study. Olanzapine yielded similar decreases in YMRS scores in patients with manic versus mixed episodes and in patients with versus those without psychotic features. Olanzapine adverse effects included somno-

·nce and weight gain (+2.1 kg with olanzapine versus +0.45 kg with placebo), with 3.6% discontinuing due to adverse events (versus 1.7% with placebo).

As noted earlier, two multicenter, randomized, double-blind, active-comparator trials (Tohen et al. 2002a; Zajecka et al. 2002) suggested that olanzapine was slightly more effective for the treatment of acute mania compared with divalproex but had slightly more adverse effects. In addition, a 12-week, multicenter, randomized, double-blind, active-comparator, acute mania trial (Tohen et al. 2003) assessed olanzapine monotherapy (started at 15 mg/day, mean week-12 dosage 11.4 mg/day) compared with haloperidol monotherapy (started at 10 mg/day, mean week-12 dosage 5.2 mg/day). The 234 patients given olanzapine—compared with 219 patients given haloperidol—had similar YMRS response and remission (YMRS less than or equal to 12; 21-item Hamilton Rating Scale for Depression less than or equal to 6) rates at 6 and 12 weeks but longer time to emergence of post-mania depression. Olanzapine yielded fewer extrapyramidal adverse effects and numerically fewer adverse event discontinuations compared with haloperidol (8.1% versus 11.4%) but produced more weight gain (2.82 versus 0.02 kg).

In a pooled analysis of two 6-week, multicenter, randomized, double-blind, placebo-controlled acute mania studies, olanzapine or placebo was added to at least 2 weeks of lithium (mean serum concentration 0.76 mEq/L) or valproate (mean serum concentration 64 µg/mL) monotherapy in patients with inadequate responses (Tohen et al. 2002b). Olanzapine was started at 10 mg/day, with a mean modal dosage of 10.4 mg/day. The YMRS response rate was greater in 220 patients given combination therapy (68%) than in 114 patients given mood stabilizer monotherapy (45%), and the mean time to response was shorter with olanzapine plus mood stabilizer (18 days) than with mood stabilizer alone (28 days). Combination treatment yielded more somnolence, dry mouth, tremor, slurred speech, increased appetite, and weight gain (3.04 kg versus 0.23 kg) and significantly more discontinuations due to adverse events (10.9% versus 1.7%) than monotherapy.

Olanzapine is available in an intramuscular formulation indicated for the treatment of agitation associated with schizophrenia and bipolar I mania. In a multicenter, randomized, double-blind, placebo-controlled trial, agitated acute mania inpatients received intramuscular olanzapine (10 mg, first two injections; 5 mg, third injection), lorazepam (2 mg, first two injections; 1 mg, third injection), or placebo (placebo, first two injections; olanzapine, 10 mg, third injection) within a 24-hour period (Meehan et al. 2001). About half of the patients were already receiving lithium or valproate. At 2 and 24 hours after the first injection, the 99 patients given olanzapine had significantly greater decreases in mean Positive and Negative Syndrome Scale–Excited Component scores compared with the 51 patients given lorazepam and the 51 patients given placebo. Somnolence (olanzapine 13%, lorazepam 10%, placebo 6%) and dizziness (olanzapine 9%, lorazepam 14%, placebo 2%) were the most common adverse events.

In acute mania, oral olanzapine as monotherapy is started at 10–15 mg/day and titrated as high as 20 mg/day. When combined with lithium or divalproex, olanzapine is started at 10 mg once a day and titrated to 5–20 mg/day. The recommended intramuscular olanzapine dosage is 10 mg (lower dosages may be considered as clinically indicated), and can be repeated after 2 hours (as necessary and tolerated) and again after 4 more hours for a maximum dosage of 30 mg/day. The most common adverse effects with oral olanzapine are somnolence, dry mouth, dizziness, asthenia, constipation, dyspepsia, increased appetite, and tremor. Somnolence is the most common adverse effect with intramuscular olanzapine. Maximal dosing of intramuscular olanzapine may yield substantial orthostatic hypotension; thus, administration of additional doses to patients with clinically significant postural changes in systolic blood pressure is not recommended. The FDA has stipulated changes in the olanzapine product information to reflect the risk of hyperglycemia and diabetes mellitus, and the report of a recent consensus development conference suggested the risks of obesity, diabetes, and hyperlipidemia with this agent (and clozapine) are greater than with other newer antipsychotics (American Diabetes Association et al. 2004). Thus, clinical and (as indicated) laboratory monitoring for obesity, diabetes, and hyperlipidemia appears prudent for patients receiving olanzapine. Other warnings in the product information include the risks of cerebrovascular adverse events, including stroke, in elderly patients with dementia, neuroleptic malignant syndrome, and tardive dyskinesia. To date, olanzapine has not been associated with congenital malformations in humans (FDA Pregnancy Category C).

Olanzapine has some drug–drug interactions, as certain enzyme inducers such as carbamazepine can decrease, and some enzyme inhibitors such as fluvoxamine may increase, serum olanzapine concentrations.

Risperidone

Risperidone received FDA approval for the short-term treatment of acute manic or mixed episodes associated with bipolar disorder as monotherapy and in combination with lithium or valproate in 2003. The first multicenter, double-blind, placebo-controlled monotherapy acute mania study (Hirschfeld et al. 2003b) was a 3-week trial in which the YMRS response rate was greater in 127 patients given risperidone (43%) than in 119 patients given placebo (24%). Risperidone compared with placebo yielded a significantly greater mean YMRS decrease by day 3. Risperidone dosages were 3 mg on day 1, 2–4 mg on day 2, 1–5 mg on day 3, and 1–6 mg on day 4 and thereafter, with a mean modal dosage of 4.4 mg/day. Risperidone adverse effects included extrapyramidal symptoms, hyperprolactinemia, and weight gain (+1.6 kg with risperidone versus –0.25 kg with placebo), with 8% discontinuing due to adverse events (versus 6% with placebo).

The second multicenter, double-blind, placebo-controlled monotherapy acute mania study (Khanna et al. 2003) was a 3-week trial in which the YMRS response rate was greater in 146 patients given risperidone (73%) than in 144 patients given placebo (36%). Risperidone compared with placebo yielded a significantly greater mean YMRS decrease by day 7. Risperidone was initiated as in the first study, with a mean modal dosage of 5.6 mg/day, and adverse effects included extrapyramidal symptoms, tremor, insomnia, somnolence, and headache. Discontinuation due to adverse events occurred in 0.7% of patients given risperidone and 1.4% of patients given placebo.

In a 3-week, multicenter, randomized, double-blind, placebo-controlled acute mania study (Sachs et al. 2002), risperidone, haloperidol, or placebo was combined with lithium or valproate. Risperidone dosages were 2 mg on days 1 and 2, 1–4 mg on days 3 and 4, and 1–6 mg/day thereafter, with a mean modal dosage of 3.8 mg/day. Haloperidol dosages were 4 mg on days 1 and 2, 2–8 mg on days 3 and 4, and 2–12 mg/day thereafter, with a mean modal dosage of 6.2 mg/day. The YMRS response rate tended to be greater among the 52 patients given risperidone plus mood stabilizer combination therapy (57%) and among the 53 patients given haloperidol plus mood stabilizer combination therapy (58%) than among the 51 patients given mood stabilizer monotherapy (38%). Both active treatments yielded similar decreases in YMRS scores in patients with manic compared with mixed episodes and in patients with versus those without psychotic features. Compared with monotherapy, risperidone plus mood stabilizer combination treatment yielded more weight gain (+5.3 lb versus +0.3 lb), and haloperidol plus mood stabilizer combination treatment yielded more extrapyramidal symptoms. Discontinuation due to adverse events occurred in 4% of those given the risperidone combination, 2% of those given the haloperidol combination, and 4% of those given mood stabilizer monotherapy.

In yet another 3-week, multicenter, randomized, double-blind, placebo-controlled acute mania study (Yatham et al. 2003), risperidone or placebo was combined with lithium, valproate, or carbamazepine. Risperidone dosages were 3 mg on days 1 and 2, 1–4 mg on days 3 and 4, and 1–6 mg/day thereafter, with a mean modal dosage of 4.0 mg/day. The YMRS response rate was greater in 75 patients given combination therapy (59%) than in 75 patients given mood stabilizer monotherapy (41%). However, carbamazepine decreased serum risperidone plus active metabolite concentrations by 40%, interfering with efficacy. Combination therapy yielded similar YMRS decreases in patients with versus those without psychotic features. Combination treatment compared to monotherapy yielded more extrapyramidal symptoms and weight gain (+1.7 kg versus +0.5 kg) but numerically fewer discontinuations due to adverse events (1% versus 4%).

In acute mania, risperidone is started at 2–3 mg once per day and adjusted by 1 mg/day as necessary and tolerated, within a range of 1–6 mg/day. The most common risperidone adverse effects with monotherapy are somnolence, dystonia, akathisia, dyspepsia, nausea, parkinsonism, blurred vision, and increased salivation; with adjunctive therapy the most common adverse effects are somnolence, dizziness, parkinsonism, increased salivation, akathisia, abdominal pain, and urinary incontinence. Risperidone also causes hyperprolactinemia that can manifest as menstrual irregularities, galactorrhea, and difficulties with sexual desire and function. The FDA has stipulated changes in the risperidone product information to reflect the risks of hyperglycemia and diabetes mellitus, and the report of a recent consensus development conference (American Diabetes Association et al. 2004) suggested the risks of obesity, diabetes, and hyperlipidemia with this agent are intermediate, being less than with clozapine and olanzapine but greater than with ziprasidone and aripiprazole. Thus, clinical and (as indicated) laboratory monitoring for obesity, diabetes, and hyperlipidemia appear prudent for patients receiving risperidone. Other warnings in the product information include the risks of cerebrovascular adverse events, including stroke, in elderly patients with dementia, neuroleptic malignant syndrome, and tardive dyskinesia. To date, risperidone has not been associated with congenital malformations in humans (FDA Pregnancy Category C).

Risperidone has some drug–drug interactions, as certain enzyme inducers such as carbamazepine can decrease serum risperidone concentrations.

Quetiapine

In 2004 quetiapine received FDA approval for the treatment of acute manic episodes associated with bipolar disorder either as monotherapy or as adjunctive therapy to lithium or divalproex. Patients with rapid cycling and mixed episodes were not included in the pivotal acute mania studies, so the efficacy of quetiapine in these subtypes remains to be established.

In multicenter, randomized, double-blind, placebo-controlled monotherapy acute mania trials quetiapine compared with placebo yielded a significantly greater mean YMRS decreases by days 4–7 and remained superior at weeks 3 and 12. In one monotherapy study (McIntyre et al., in review), at week 3, YMRS response rates for 102 patients given quetiapine (43%) and for 98 patients given haloperidol (56%) were significantly greater than in 100 patients given placebo (35%), with a similar finding at week 12 (quetiapine 61%, haloperidol 70%, placebo 39%). Quetiapine compared with placebo yielded significantly more weight gain than placebo (+0.9 kg versus –0.3 kg) and tended to cause more somnolence and postural hypotension. Haloperidol compared with placebo had significantly greater extrapyramidal symptoms, akathisia, and tremor. Discontinuation due to adverse events was noted in 4.9% of patients given quetiapine, 10.1% given haloperidol, and 5.9% given placebo.

In another 12-week acute mania study (Bowden et al. 2005), YMRS response rate at week 3 in 107 patients given quetiapine (53%) was similar to that in 98 patients given lithium (53%) and significantly exceeded that of 95 patients given placebo (27%). At week 12, quetiapine (72%) and lithium (76%) response rates still exceeded that of placebo (41%). Quetiapine compared with placebo yielded dry mouth, somnolence, weight gain (+2.63 kg versus –0.08 kg), and dizziness, with 6.5% discontinuing due to adverse events versus 4.1% with placebo and 6.1% with lithium.

In a pooled analysis of the two monotherapy studies just discussed, quetiapine compared with placebo yielded a significantly greater mean YMRS decrease by day 4, and this persisted through day 84 (Calabrese et al., in review).

In a 3-week, multicenter, randomized, double-blind, placebo-controlled acute mania trial (Sachs et al. 2004a), YMRS response rate of 91 patients given quetiapine combined with lithium or divalproex (54%) exceeded that of 100 patients given mood stabilizer monotherapy (33%). Combination compared with monotherapy yielded more somnolence, dry mouth, asthenia, postural hypotension, and weight gain (1.6 kg versus 0.36 kg), but numerically fewer adverse event discontinuations (5.5% versus 6.0%). In a pooled analysis of this trial and a similar 6-week study, the YMRS response rate at week 3 for 185 patients given quetiapine plus mood stabilizer (56%) exceeded that of 185 patients given mood stabilizer monotherapy (42%) (Yatham et al. 2004). Combination compared with monotherapy yielded a significantly greater mean YMRS decrease by day 7, which was also evident at days 14 and 21. Combination compared with monotherapy yielded more somnolence, dry mouth, asthenia, postural hypotension, and weight gain (1.97 kg versus 0.27 kg) but fewer adverse event discontinuations by day 21 (3.0% versus 3.9%).

In these studies, quetiapine dosage was 100 mg on day 1, 200 mg on day 2, 300 mg on day 3, 400 mg on day 4, up to 600 mg on day 5, and up to 800 mg thereafter. Mean final quetiapine dosages were approximately 430–500 mg/day for monotherapy and about 430–575 mg/day for adjunctive therapy. This approach is thus the recommended regimen in the product information.

Finally, in a small 6-week, randomized, double-blind, placebo-controlled adolescent acute mania trial (Delbello et al. 2002), the YMRS response rate of 15 patients given quetiapine combined with divalproex (87%) exceeded that of 15 patients given divalproex monotherapy (53%). Quetiapine was started at 50 mg/day and titrated, with a mean dosage of 432 mg/day. Divalproex was started at 20 mg/kg/day and titrated, with mean serum concentrations of 102 and 104 µg/mL in the monotherapy and combination therapy groups, respectively. Combination compared with monotherapy yielded more sedation.

The most common adverse events with quetiapine are somnolence, dizziness (postural hypotension), dry mouth, constipation, increased serum glutamate pyruvate transaminase, weight gain, and dyspepsia. The FDA has stipulated changes in the quetiapine product information to reflect the risks of hyperglycemia and diabetes mellitus, and the report of a recent consensus development conference (American Diabetes Association et al. 2004) suggested the risks of obesity, diabetes, and hyperlipidemia with this agent are intermediate, being less than with clozapine and olanzapine but more than with ziprasidone and aripiprazole. Thus, clinical and (as indicated) laboratory monitoring for obesity, diabetes, and hyperlipidemia appear prudent for patients receiving quetiapine. Other warnings in the product information include the risks of neuroleptic malignant syndrome and tardive dyskinesia. To date, quetiapine has not been associated with congenital malformations in humans (FDA Pregnancy Category C).

Quetiapine has some drug–drug interactions, as certain enzyme inducers such as carbamazepine can decrease, and some enzyme inhibitors such as macrolide antibiotics may increase, serum quetiapine concentrations. In addition, combining quetiapine with antiarrhythmia medications is not recommended due to the concerns regarding the potential for additive cardiac conduction delays.

Ziprasidone

Ziprasidone received FDA approval in 2004 as monotherapy for the treatment of acute manic or mixed episodes associated with bipolar disorder, with or without psychotic features. In a 3-week, multicenter, randomized, double-blind, placebo-controlled acute mania trial (Keck et al. 2003b), the YMRS response rate for 131 patients given ziprasidone monotherapy (50%) exceeded that in 66 patients given placebo (35%). Ziprasidone yielded a significantly greater mean YMRS decrease than placebo by day 2. Ziprasidone dosages (given with meals) were 40 mg twice a day on day 1, 80 mg twice a day on day 2, and thereafter titrated, with the total daily dosage between 80 mg/day and 160 mg/day and a mean daily dosage of 130 mg/day for the final week of the study. Ziprasidone adverse events included somnolence, headache, dizziness, hypertonia, nausea, and akathisia, with 6.4% of monotherapy subjects discontinuing due to adverse effects versus 4.3% of those given placebo.

In a second 3-week, multicenter, randomized, double-blind, placebo-controlled acute mania trial (Segal et al. 2004), the YMRS response rate for 137 patients given ziprasidone monotherapy (46%) exceeded that of 65 patients given placebo (29%). Again, ziprasidone compared to placebo yielded a significantly greater mean YMRS decrease by day 2. Ziprasidone was initiated as in the prior trial, with a mean daily dosage of 112 mg/day for the final week of the study. Ziprasidone adverse events included somnolence, headache, extrapyramidal symptoms, dizziness, akathisia, nausea, tremor, blurred vision, asthenia, constipation, dry mouth, and dystonia, with 6.5% of monotherapy patients discontinuing versus 1.5% of those given placebo.

In a pooled analysis of these two studies, ziprasidone monotherapy appeared to have a broad spectrum of efficacy, demonstrating comparable benefits in patients with manic versus mixed episodes and those with versus without psychotic symptoms (Potkin et al. 2004).

In a multicenter, randomized, double-blind, placebo-controlled acute mania trial (Weisler et al. 2004a), 99 patients given ziprasidone combined with open lithium versus 99 given placebo and open lithium had a significantly greater mean YMRS decrease at day 4, but only numerically greater mean YMRS decreases at days 7, 14, and 21. The authors suggested that combining ziprasidone with lithium in acute mania might accelerate response. Ziprasidone dosage was 80 mg on day 1, 160 mg on day 2, and 80–160 mg/day thereafter. Open lithium was dosed to yield serum lithium concentrations between 0.8 mEq/L and 1.2 mEq/L. Ziprasidone plus lithium versus lithium monotherapy yielded more somnolence, extrapyramidal symptoms, dizziness, agitation, and discontinuations due to adverse events (8% versus 4%).

Ziprasidone is available in an intramuscular formulation that is indicated for the treatment of acute agitation in schizophrenic patients for whom treatment with ziprasidone is appropriate and who need intramuscular antipsychotic medication for rapid control of agitation. To date, intramuscular ziprasidone has not been approved for the treatment of patients with bipolar disorder. However, the efficacy of intramuscular ziprasidone in psychotic agitated patients with bipolar disorder (manic or mixed episodes with psychotic features; BP) or schizoaffective disorder bipolar type (SABP) was assessed in a subgroup analysis of two similarly designed, 24-hour, randomized, double-blind, fixed-dose studies (Daniel et al. 2004). Intramuscular ziprasidone 10–20 mg (up to four doses in 24 hours) was compared with a ziprasidone 2 mg control (up to four doses in 24 hours). The Behavioral Activity Rating Scale response (more than 2-point decrease at 1.5 hours after first dose) rate in 15 patients (8 BP, 7 SABP) given ziprasidone 20 mg (80%) exceeded that of 11 patients (4 BP, 7 SABP) given 2 mg (18%). In 20 patients (10 BP, 10 SABP) given ziprasidone

10 mg and 15 patients (4 BP, 11 SABP) on ziprasidone 2 mg, Behavioral Activity Rating Scale response rates were 57% and 36%, respectively. One patient in the ziprasidone 10 mg group had akathisia, but no dystonia or excessive sedation was reported.

In acute mania patients, oral ziprasidone is started at 40 mg twice a day with food, increased to 60–80 mg on the second day, and subsequently adjusted as needed and tolerated within the range of 40–80 mg. Intramuscular ziprasidone requires reconstitution prior to administration and has a recommended dosage in agitation in schizophrenia of 10 mg every 2 hours (or 20 mg every 4 hours) as needed up to 40 mg/day.

The most common adverse events associated with discontinuation of ziprasidone in acute mania were akathisia, anxiety, depression, dizziness, dystonia, rash, and vomiting. The most common adverse events with intramuscular ziprasidone in schizophrenia patients were headache, nausea, and somnolence. The FDA has stipulated that the ziprasidone product information include the risks of hyperglycemia and diabetes mellitus, but the consensus development conference mentioned previously (American Diabetes Association et al. 2004) reported that the risks of obesity, diabetes, and hyperlipidemia with ziprasidone are similar to those with aripiprazole and are less than with other newer antipsychotics. Thus, clinical and (as indicated) laboratory monitoring for obesity, diabetes, and hyperlipidemia may be prudent for patients receiving ziprasidone. Other warnings in the product information include the risks of neuroleptic malignant syndrome, tardive dyskinesia, and QT prolongation and risk of sudden death. Although pre-marketing studies suggested that ziprasidone yielded cardiac conduction delays, post-marketing experience to date has failed to indicate clinically significant problems with cardiac conduction. To date, ziprasidone has not been associated with congenital malformations in humans (FDA Pregnancy Category C).

Ziprasidone has some drug–drug interactions, as certain enzyme inducers such as carbamazepine can decrease, and some enzyme inhibitors such as macrolide antibiotics may increase, serum ziprasidone concentrations. In addition, combining ziprasidone with antiarrhythmia medications is not recommended because of concerns about the potential for additive cardiac conduction delays.

Aripiprazole

Aripiprazole received FDA approval in 2004 for monotherapy treatment of acute manic or mixed episodes associated with bipolar disorder and in early 2005 received a maintenance indication. In the first 3-week, multicenter, randomized, double-blind, placebo-controlled acute mania study (Keck et al. 2003a), the YMRS response rate for 123 patients given aripiprazole monotherapy (40%) exceeded that of 120 patients given placebo (19%). Aripiprazole yielded a significantly greater mean YMRS decrease than placebo by day 4. Aripiprazole was started at 30 mg/day but could be reduced to 15 mg/day for tolerability if needed, with a mean final daily dosage of 28 mg/day. Aripiprazole adverse effects included headache, nausea, dyspepsia, vomiting, constipation, somnolence, accidental injury, and akathisia, with 11% of patients discontinuing aripiprazole due to adverse effects versus 10% with placebo.

In another 3-week, multicenter, randomized, double-blind, placebo-controlled acute mania study (Sachs et al. 2004b), the YMRS response rate for 135 patients given aripiprazole monotherapy (53%) exceeded that of 129 patients given placebo (32%). Again, aripiprazole yielded a significantly greater mean YMRS decrease by day 4. Aripiprazole was administered as in the first trial, with a mean final daily dosage of 28 mg/day. Aripiprazole adverse effects included dyspepsia, constipation, akathisia, and extremity pain, with 9% of patients discontinuing aripiprazole due to adverse effects versus 7% with placebo.

In a pooled analysis of three (the two above plus one additional) acute mania studies, aripiprazole monotherapy appeared to have a broad spectrum of efficacy (Jody et al. 2004). Thus, aripiprazole demonstrated comparable benefits in patients with more severe (baseline YMRS score greater than 28) versus less severe (baseline YMRS score less than 28) mania, with manic versus mixed episodes, with versus without psychotic symptoms, and with versus without rapid cycling.

In a 12-week, multicenter, randomized, double-blind, active-comparator acute mania trial, 173 patients given aripiprazole and 164 patients given haloperidol had similar decreases in YMRS scores at the end of weeks 3 and 12 (Vieta et al., in press). Patients with a Clinical Global Impression–Bipolar Disorder mania score greater than 4 or a Montgomery-Åsberg Depression Rating Scale score greater than 18 at the end of week 3 were discontinued from the study. Overall, 51% of patients given aripiprazole and 29% given haloperidol completed the study. In an analysis that considered patients not completing the trial to be nonresponders, the YMRS response rate at the end of week 12 in patients given aripiprazole (50%) exceeded that in patients given haloperidol (28%). Aripiprazole was started at 15 mg/day, with the option to increase to 30 mg/day, and a mean week 12 dosage of 22 mg/day. Haloperidol was started at 10 mg/day, with the option to increase to 15 mg/day, and a mean week 12 dosage of 11 mg/day. Aripiprazole compared with haloperidol yielded fewer extrapyramidal symptoms and akathisia. Other adverse events observed with both agents included tremor, headache, depression, and insomnia.

Perhaps due to partial agonist effects at dopamine receptors, nausea and vomiting can occur if aripiprazole is started at higher dosages (such as 30 mg/day). Gastrointestinal tolerability is enhanced in acute mania patients if aripiprazole is initiated at 15 mg/day or lower for a few days before increasing to 30 mg/day. The FDA has stipulated that the aripiprazole product information include the risks of hyperglycemia and diabetes mellitus, but the consensus development conference report (American Diabetes Association et al. 2004) suggested the risks of obesity, diabetes, and hyperlipidemia with aripiprazole are similar to those with ziprasidone and less than with other newer antipsychotics. Thus, clinical and (as indicated) laboratory monitoring for obesity, diabetes, and hyperlipidemia may be prudent for patients receiving aripiprazole. Other warnings in the product information include the risks of cerebrovascular adverse events, including stroke, in elderly patients with dementia, neuroleptic malignant syndrome, and tardive dyskinesia. To date, aripiprazole has not been associated with congenital malformations in humans (FDA Pregnancy Category C).

Aripiprazole has some drug–drug interactions, as enzyme inducers such as carbamazepine can decrease, and some enzyme inhibitors such as macrolide antibiotics may increase, serum aripiprazole concentrations.

Newer Anticonvulsants

The efficacy and tolerability limitations of lithium and antipsychotics and the utility of valproate and carbamazepine in bipolar disorders resulted in the assessment of several of newer anticonvulsants in acute mania. These newer anticonvulsants appear to have diverse psychotropic profiles. Although not generally effective for acute mania (with the possible exception of oxcarbazepine; see Table 2–1), these medications may have utility for other aspects of bipolar disorders (such as lamotrigine for maintenance or acute bipolar depression) or comorbid conditions.

Table 2–1. New anticonvulsants not (yet) proven effective in mania

Drug	Evidence
Oxcarbazepine	Underpowered active-comparator monotherapy studies (Emrich 1990)
Gabapentin	Negative placebo-controlled adjunctive study (Pande et al. 2000a)
Lamotrigine	Negative placebo- and lithium-controlled adjunctive study (Bowden et al. 2000)
Topiramate	Negative placebo- and lithium-controlled adult monotherapy studies (Powers et al. 2004)
Tiagabine	Negative open adjunctive study (Grunze et al. 1999)
Levetiracetam	No controlled study
Zonisamide	No controlled study
Benzodiazepines	Underpowered active-comparator monotherapy study (Bradwejn et al. 1990)
	Common adjuncts that do not interfere with separation of active treatments from placebo

Oxcarbazepine

Oxcarbazepine, a cogener of carbamazepine, may differ from other newer anticonvulsants in that, like carbamazepine and valproate, it may have efficacy in acute mania. Oxcarbazepine's structural similarity to carbamazepine suggests the possibility that oxcarbazepine could have psychotropic effects that overlap those of carbamazepine, and as noted later, oxcarbazepine compared with carbamazepine has more favorable adverse effect and drug interaction profiles. Unfortunately, there is very little evidence of efficacy for oxcarbazepine in bipolar disorders, far less than for carbamazepine. Specifically, to date, there are no large double-blind, placebo-controlled trials of oxcarbazepine in bipolar disorders.

In an early, small, double-blind, on-off-on trial in six patients (Emrich et al. 1983), oxcarbazepine 1,800 to 2,100 mg/day yielded about a 50% decrease in mania ratings. In a small, multicenter, active-comparator 15-day acute mania study, 19 patients given oxcarbazepine (mean dosage 2,400 mg/day) had improvement similar to that seen in 19 patients given haloperidol (mean dosage 42 mg/day), and in a similar study 28 patients given oxcarbazepine (mean dosage 1,400 mg/day) had improvement similar to that in 24 patients given lithium (mean dosage 1,100 mg/day) (Emrich 1990). Oxcarbazepine was generally well tolerated in all of these studies. Methodological limitations included the lack of placebo control and the use of small samples that markedly limited statistical power.

Based on generally better tolerability and fewer drug interactions (compared with carbamazepine), oxcarbazepine has been proposed as an alternative intervention for acute mania and maintenance treatment in bipolar disorders (American Psychiatric Association 2002). However, larger double-blind, placebo-controlled studies are necessary to determine whether oxcarbazepine is effective in bipolar disorders.

Oxcarbazepine dosages are about 50% higher than those used with carbamazepine, often starting at 300–600 mg/day and increasing by 300 mg/day every few days as necessary and tolerated to maximum dosages of 900–2,400 mg/day. Serum concentrations range between 10 and 35 μg/mL. The latter values are derived from usage in epilepsy, and oxcarbazepine is generally dosed clinically in bipolar disorders, titrating to desired effect as tolerated.

Oxcarbazepine appears to be generally better tolerated than carbamazepine, yielding less neurotoxicity and rash (Friis et al. 1993). Oxcarbazepine has not been associated with blood dyscrasias, lacks a "black-box" warning in the product information, and does not appear to require hematological monitoring. Warnings in the product information include the 25% chance of cross-hypersensitivity with carbamazepine and the risk of hyponatremia. Hyponatremia may be the main adverse effect that occurs more commonly with oxcarbazepine than with carbamazepine (Isojarvi et al. 2001). Oxcarbazepine, like carbamazepine, may yield transaminase elevations and gastrointestinal adverse effects but has less weight gain than valproate (Rattya et al. 1999). Oxcarbazepine, in contrast to carbamazepine, has not to date been associated with congenital malformations in humans (FDA Pregnancy Category C). However, this could be related to fewer oxcarbazepine exposures.

Oxcarbazepine has generally fewer drug–drug interactions than carbamazepine. Unlike carbamazepine, oxcarbazepine does not yield autoinduction of metabolism, and its metabolism is not susceptible to enzyme inhibitors. Thus, addition of other drugs does not tend to increase oxcarbazepine blood concentrations. Also, oxcarbazepine (compared with carbamazepine) appears to have less robust heteroinduction. Hence, unlike with carbamazepine, dosage adjustment of some other medications such as lamotrigine or valproate in patients receiving oxcarbazepine is not recommended. However, oxcarbazepine appears to have a clinically significant interaction with hormonal contraceptives, decreasing blood concentrations by up to about 50% (Fattore et al. 1999).

Lamotrigine

Unlike divalproex and carbamazepine, lamotrigine does *not* appear to be effective in acute mania. In two multicenter, randomized, double-blind, placebo-controlled studies, lamotrigine was no more effective than placebo in acute mania (Bowden et al. 2000). One of these was a failed 3-week low-dose study in which antipsychotics were allowed for the first 5 days, with SAD-C Mania Rating Scale response rates that were similar for 85 patients given lamotrigine (final dosage 50 mg/day) (44%), 95 patients given placebo (46%), and 36 given lithium (42%). The other report was a 6-week add-on (antipsychotics were allowed up to week 3) study in which the response rate in 77 patients given lithium (62%) was significantly higher than in 77 given placebo (47%), whereas the response in 77 patients given lamotrigine (final dosage 200 mg/day; 55%) failed to achieve statistical separation from placebo. In these studies, although lamotrigine did not significantly decrease SAD-C Mania Rating Scale scores, it also did not appear to cause exacerbation of mania, because there were similar percentages of patients with increases for lamotrigine, lithium, and placebo.

In contrast, double-blind, placebo-controlled studies have found lamotrigine effective in maintenance treatment (particularly for preventing depressive episodes) of bipolar I disorder (Bowden et al. 2003; Calabrese et al. 2003). Thus, as described in Chapter 4, lamotrigine received an FDA indication for maintenance treatment in bipolar I disorder to delay the time to occurrence of mood episodes (depression, mania, hypomania, mixed episodes) in patients treated for acute mood episodes with standard therapy. Also, as described by Sachs (Chapter 3), controlled data suggest lamotrigine is effective in acute bipolar depression (Calabrese et al. 1999) as well as in rapid-cycling bipolar disorder (a depression-predominant subtype of bipolar disorder; Calabrese et al. 2000), and in treatment-resistant (primarily rapid-cycling bipolar) mood disorders (Frye et al. 2000), as Chapter 5 details.

Hence, lamotrigine may "stabilize mood from below" in the sense that it may maximally impact depressive symptoms in bipolar disorders (Ketter and Calabrese 2002). In contrast, the older mood stabilizers (lithium, carbamazepine, and valproate) and at least some newer antipsychotics appear to "stabilize mood from above" in that they may maximally impact manic or hypomanic symptoms in bipolar disorders.

Despite its inefficacy for acute mania, use of lamotrigine may be considered once standard therapy for acute mania has commenced, with the goal of preventing or delaying a post-mania depression. Although controlled data are limited, observations from the open stabilization phase of a maintenance trial in bipolar I disorder patients who were currently or recently (within prior 2 months) manic or hypomanic are worth noting (Bowden et al. 2003). In this study, open addition of lamotrigine to standard therapies allowed 175 of 349 (50%) patients to stabilize sufficiently (Clinical Global Impression Scale score of 3 or less for 4 weeks) within 8–16 weeks (despite tapering off other medications) to be randomized for the controlled maintenance trial. This intervention was generally well tolerated. This approach has the strength of achieving full dosage of lamotrigine sooner, which is particularly desirable given the gradual initial titration of lamotrigine. Limitations include potential adverse effects and drug interactions related to introduction of a medication not directly targeting mood elevation during acute mania. For example, as noted in Chapters 4 and 5, concurrent valproate may increase the risk of the common (1 in 10) benign and rare (1 in 1,000) serious rashes associated with lamotrigine, and valproate doubles and carbamazepine halves serum lamotrigine concentrations, requiring lamotrigine dosage adjustments. In addition, occasional patients may experience activation with lamotrigine. However, as noted earlier, in two controlled studies there were similar percentages of patients with SAD-C Mania Rating Scale score increases for lamotrigine, lithium, and placebo (Bowden et al. 2000), suggesting that activation may be a sporadic occurrence—certainly of clinical significance in patients in whom it has been observed, but not a significant population-wide effect that would generally contraindicate introducing lamotrigine once standard therapy has commenced. Taken together, these studies indicate that the strengths and limitations of adding lamotrigine once standard therapy begins need to be carefully considered on a patient-by-patient basis prior to embarking upon such an intervention. Additional controlled trials would help to better inform clinicians regarding this issue.

Gabapentin

Although early open reports of gabapentin use in bipolar disorders were encouraging, later randomized, double-blind, placebo-controlled studies were discouraging. Thus, in outpatients with acute mania or hypomania despite treatment with lithium or valproate, gabapentin 600–3,600 mg/day was no better than adding placebo (Pande et al. 2000a). Also, in treatment-resistant (mainly rapid-cycling bipolar) mood disorder inpatients, gabapentin monotherapy at a dosage of 4,000 mg/day was no better than placebo (Frye et al. 2000). In view of the absence of controlled data supporting efficacy in mania, gabapentin was *not* considered to be an option in the management of mania when the practice guideline was revised in 2002 (American Psychiatric Association 2002). In contrast, gabapentin appeared effective in several comorbid conditions seen in patients with bipolar disorders, with double-blind, placebo-controlled trials demonstrating efficacy in anxiety disorders such as social phobia (Pande et al. 1999) and (in a post-hoc analysis) moderate to severe panic disorder (Pande et al. 2000b) and in pain syndromes such as neuropathic pain (Serpell 2002), chronic daily headache (Spira and Beran 2003), and post-herpetic neuralgia (for which it was given an FDA indication; Rowbotham et al. 1998).

Topiramate

Although early open reports of topiramate in bipolar disorders were encouraging, later multicenter, randomized, double-blind, placebo-controlled studies were discouraging. Thus, in several trials topiramate proved no better or worse than placebo in adults with acute mania (Powers et al. 2004). Thus topiramate was *not* considered an option in the management of mania in the practice guideline revision (American Psychiatric Association 2002). However, in a 4-week, multicenter, randomized, double-blind, placebo-controlled adolescent acute mania trial (DelBello et al. 2004), 29 adolescents given topiramate (mean dosage 278 mg/day) compared with 27 given placebo had a significantly greater mean YMRS decrease at day 28. However, this study was terminated early when the adult acute mania trials failed to show efficacy. Additional evaluation of topiramate in acute mania in adolescents may be warranted.

Topiramate appeared effective in several comorbid conditions seen in patients with bipolar disorders, with randomized, double-blind, placebo-controlled trials demonstrating efficacy in eating disorders such as bulimia (Hoopes et al. 2003), binge eating disorder with obesity (McElroy et al. 2003), and obesity (Bray et al. 2003), as well as in alcohol dependence (Johnson et al. 2003) and the prevention of migraine headaches (Brandes et al. 2004). Weight loss has consistently been observed in controlled trials with topiramate, not only in patients with eating disorders but also in manic (Powers et al. 2004) and depressed (McIntyre et al. 2002) patients with bipolar disorders.

Tiagabine

There are no controlled studies of tiagabine in bipolar disorders. Although some experience with open low-dose tiagabine in bipolar disorders has been encouraging (Schaffer et al. 2002), other open reports have suggested problems with both efficacy and tolerability. For example, rapid loading of open, primarily adjunctive tiagabine starting at 20 mg/day (five times the recommended starting dosage) in eight inpatients with acute mania was not only ineffective but also yielded unacceptable adverse effects, with one patient having a seizure (Grunze et al. 1999). This suggests not only inefficacy in mania but also that loading or rapid dosage escalation should be avoided and caution exercised in using tiagabine, particularly in the initial titration phase. However, even more gradual initiation may be problematic. Thus, open, primarily adjunctive tiagabine initiated at 4 mg/day and increased weekly as tolerated by 4 mg/day (mean dosage 8.7 mg/day, mean duration 38 days) in 13 outpatients with treatment-refractory bipolar disorder (7 depressed, 6 hypomanic) had limited efficacy, with 10 of 13 (77%) patients having no change or worsening of clinical symptoms, and raised tolerability concerns because 2 of 13 (15%) patients had seizures attributed as likely due to the medication (Suppes et al. 2002). Thus, open studies have raised both efficacy and tolerability concerns regarding tiagabine in bipolar disorders. In contrast, small controlled trials have reported that low-dose (less than 16 mg/day) tiagabine was generally well tolerated and yielded benefit in generalized anxiety disorder (Rosenthal 2003) and primary insomnia (Roth and Walsh 2004). Taken together, these data suggest that like gabapentin and topiramate, tiagabine does not appear to be effective as a primary treatment for bipolar disorders but may yield benefit in common comorbid problems (such as generalized anxiety disorders and insomnia). However, reports of tolerability problems suggest that considerable caution ought to be exercised with this agent in patients with bipolar disorders (Grunze et al. 1999; Suppes et al. 2002).

Levetiracetam

To date there are no controlled studies and only a few open reports regarding levetiracetam effects in bipolar disorders (Goldberg and Burdick 2002). In 10 acute mania inpatients, open levetiracetam added to haloperidol 5–10 mg/day starting at 1,000 mg/day and titrated over 4 days to as high as 4,000 mg/day (mean dosage 3,125 mg/day) decreased YMRS scores in an on-off-on design (Grunze et al. 2003). Dosing in this study was more aggressive than the recommended epilepsy regimen of starting with 1,000 mg/day and increasing every 2 weeks by 1,000 mg/day as tolerated, with a maximum recommended dosage of 3,000 mg/day. Despite the aggressive titration in this acute mania study, open adjunctive levetiracetam was generally well tolerated and yielded only sedation, dizziness, and asthenia in a few patients (Grunze et al. 2003). These data suggest that systematic evaluation of levetiracetam's potential for utility in bipolar disorders is needed.

Zonisamide

To date there are no controlled studies and only a few open reports regarding the efficacy of zonisamide in bipolar disorders. In a small open treatment study, addition of zonisamide (mean dosage 280 mg/day in bipolar patients) in 24 patients (15 bipolar disorder, manic; 6 schizoaffective disorder, bipolar type, manic; and 3 schizophrenia with agitation) significantly decreased mania ratings with response (more than moderate improvement on Clinical Psychopharmacology Rating Scale) rates of 71% in all patients and 80% in those with bipolar disorder (Kanba et al. 1994). However, based on a response criterion of a 50% decrease in Clinical Psychopharmacology Rating Scale scores, only 5 of 15 (33%) bipolar patients responded.

Emerging evidence suggests that zonisamide, like topiramate, may have utility in obesity and eating disorders. In a double-blind, placebo-controlled trial, zonisamide yielded weight loss in obesity patients (Gadde et al. 2003), and in an open trial, zonisamide offered benefit in binge eating disorder (McElroy et al. 2004). Another study suggested that open adjunctive zonisamide, starting with 100 mg/day at bedtime and increasing by 100 mg/day every 2 weeks as tolerated with a target of 300–600 mg/day (mean dosage about 450 mg/day), might yield weight loss in obese euthymic medicated patients with bipolar disorder (Yang et al. 2003).

Benzodiazepines

Benzodiazepines may have modest antimanic activity. In a small (24-patient), 2-week, double-blind acute mania study (Bradwejn et al. 1990), lorazepam and clonazepam monotherapy yielded response rates of 61% and 18%, respectively. However, the modest degree of benefit with benzodiazepines is demonstrated by experience derived from their common use as adjunctive medications early in the randomized phase of controlled trials of other agents in acute mania. Typically, in such trials, an agent such as lorazepam is permitted as needed for insomnia, anxiety, or agitation, starting at approximately 4–6 mg/day and tapering to zero over about the first week. Although this intervention may attenuate some symptoms (such as insomnia or anxiety) encountered in patients with acute mania, it does not appear to robustly attenuate the manic syndrome or systematically interfere with the ability to separate active treatments from placebo, consistent with benzodiazepines having at most modest antimanic effects.

However, the hypnotic (Andersen and Lingjaerde 1969) and anxiolytic (Ballenger et al. 1988) actions of benzodiazepines can prove clinically beneficial in patients with bipolar disorders, because insomnia and anxiety are commonly encountered symptoms. For example, up to 20% of patients with bipolar disorders may also have panic disorder (MacKinnon et al. 2002). Thus, like gabapentin and topiramate, although benzodiazepines do not appear to be effective as primary treatments for bipolar disorders, they may yield benefit in common comorbid problems (such as anxiety disorders and insomnia).

Benzodiazepines are generally well tolerated but can cause sedation and ataxia, especially when combined with other agents with such effects. Benzodiazepines appear to be associated with minor congenital malformations (FDA Pregnancy Category D). In addition, the utility of these agents is limited by their abuse potential (particularly in patients with histories of substance abuse) and the risk of disinhibition (particularly in children and adolescents and patients with Cluster B personality disorders).

Conclusions

Recent clinical trials have not only helped us better understand the utility of older agents like lithium, valproate, and carbamazepine but also have provided clinicians with additional options for the management of acute mania. Newer antipsychotics and newer anticonvulsants are the two main groups of agents that have been investigated, and they have important differences. Newer antipsychotics generally appear effective for acute mania but may differ from one another with respect to adverse effects. In contrast, newer anticonvulsants have diverse psychotropic profiles, and although not generally effective for acute mania (with the possible exception of oxcarbazepine), they may have utility for other aspects of bipolar disorders or for comorbid conditions. Additional clinical studies of these newer antipsychotics and newer anticonvulsants promise to yield further new insights into the pathophysiology and treatment of acute mania.

References

Alsdorf RM, Wyszynski DF, et al: Evidence of increased birth defects in the offspring of women exposed to valproate during pregnancy: findings from the AED pregnancy registry. Birth Defects Res: Clin Mol Ter 70:245, 2004

American Diabetes Association, American Psychiatric Association, American Association of Clinical Endocrinologists, et al: Consensus development conference on antipsychotic drugs and obesity and diabetes. Diabetes Care 27:596–601, 2004

American Psychiatric Association: Practice guideline for the treatment of patients with bipolar disorder (revision). Am J Psychiatry 159:1–50, 2002

Altshuler LL, Rasgon NL, Saad M, et al: Reproductive endocrine function in women treated for bipolar disorder. Presented at the 157th annual meeting of the American Psychiatric Association, New York, May 2004

Andersen T, Lingjaerde O: Nitrazepam (Mogadon) as a sleep-inducing agent: an analysis based on a double-blind comparison with phenobarbitone. Br J Psychiatry 115:1393–1397, 1969

Ballenger JC, Burrows GD, DuPont RL Jr, et al: Alprazolam in panic disorder and agoraphobia: results from a multicenter trial, I: efficacy in short-term treatment. Arch Gen Psychiatry 45:413–422, 1988

Bourin M, Auby P, Marcus RN, et al: Aripiprazole versus haloperidol for maintained treatment effect in acute mania. Presented at the 156th annual meeting of the American Psychiatric Association, San Francisco, CA, May 2003

Bowden CL, Brugger AM, Swann AC, et al: Efficacy of divalproex vs. lithium and placebo in the treatment of mania: The Depakote Mania Study Group. JAMA 271:918–924, 1994

Bowden CL, Janicak PG, Orsulak P, et al: Relation of serum valproate concentration to response in mania. Am J Psychiatry 153:765–770, 1996

Bowden C, Calabrese J, Ascher J, et al: Spectrum of efficacy of lamotrigine in bipolar disorder: overview of double-blind placebo-controlled studies. Presented at the 39th annual meeting of the American College of Neuropsychopharmacology. San Juan, Puerto Rico, December 2000

Bowden CL, Calabrese JR, Sachs G, et al: A placebo-controlled 18-month trial of lamotrigine and lithium maintenance treatment in recently manic or hypomanic patients with bipolar I disorder. Arch Gen Psychiatry 60:392–400, 2003

Bowden CL, Grunze H, Mullen J, et al: A randomized, double-blind, placebo-controlled efficacy and safety study of quetiapine or lithium as monotherapy for mania in bipolar disorder. J Clin Psychiatry 66:111–121, 2005

Bradwejn J, Shriqui C, Koszycki D, et al: Double-blind comparison of the effects of clonazepam and lorazepam in acute mania. J Clin Psychopharmacol 10:403–408, 1990

Brandes JL, Saper JR, Diamond M, et al: Topiramate for migraine prevention: a randomized controlled trial. JAMA 291:965–973, 2004

Bray GA, Hollander P, Klein S, et al: A 6-month randomized, placebo-controlled, dose-ranging trial of topiramate for weight loss in obesity. Obes Res 11:722–733, 2003

Calabrese JR, Bowden CL, Sachs GS, et al: Lamictal 602 Study Group: a double-blind placebo-controlled study of lamotrigine monotherapy in outpatients with bipolar I depression. J Clin Psychiatry 60:79–88, 1999

Calabrese JR, Suppes T, Bowden CL, et al: Lamictal 614 Study Group: a double-blind, placebo-controlled, prophylaxis study of lamotrigine in rapid-cycling bipolar disorder. J Clin Psychiatry 61:841–850, 2000

Calabrese JR, Bowden CL, Sachs G, et al: A placebo-controlled 18-month trial of lamotrigine and lithium maintenance treatment in recently depressed patients with bipolar I disorder. J Clin Psychiatry 64:1013–1024, 2003

Calabrese JR, Vieta E, Mullen J, et al: Quetiapine monotherapy for mania associated with bipolar disorder: analysis of two international, double-blind, randomised, placebo-controlled studies. Curr Res Med Opin, in review

Cunnington MC: The international lamotrigine pregnancy registry update for the epilepsy foundation. Epilepsia 45:1468, 2004

Daniel DG, Brook S, Warrington L, et al: Intramuscular ziprasidone in agitated psychotic patients. Presented at the 157th annual meeting of the American Psychiatric Association. New York, May 2004

Delbello MP, Schwiers ML, Rosenberg HL, et al: A double-blind, randomized, placebo-controlled study of quetiapine as adjunctive treatment for adolescent mania. J Am Acad Child Adolesc Psychiatry 41:1216–1223, 2002

DelBello MP, Kushner SF, Wang D, et al: Topiramate for acute mania in adolescent patients with bipolar I disorder. Presented at the 157th annual meeting of the American Psychiatric Association. New York, May 2004

Emrich HM: Studies with (Trileptal) oxcarbazepine in acute mania. Int Clin Psychopharmacol 5 (suppl 1):83–88, 1990

Emrich HM, Altmann H, Dose M, et al: Therapeutic effects of GABA-ergic drugs in affective disorders: a preliminary report. Pharmacol Biochem Behav 19:369–372, 1983

Fattore C, Cipolla G, Gatti G, et al: Induction of ethinylestradiol and levonorgestrel metabolism by oxcarbazepine in healthy women. Epilepsia 40:783–787, 1999

Freeman TW, Clothier JL, Pazzaglia P, et al: A double-blind comparison of valproate and lithium in the treatment of acute mania. Am J Psychiatry 149:108–111, 1992

Friis ML, Kristensen O, Boas J, et al: Therapeutic experiences with 947 epileptic outpatients in oxcarbazepine treatment. Acta Neurol Scand 87:224–227, 1993

Frye MA, Ketter TA, Altshuler LL, et al: Clozapine in bipolar disorder: treatment implications for other atypical antipsychotics. J Affect Disord 48:91–104, 1998

Frye MA, Ketter TA, Kimbrell TA, et al: A placebo-controlled study of lamotrigine and gabapentin monotherapy in refractory mood disorders. J Clin Psychopharmacol 20:607–614, 2000

Gadde KM, Franciscy DM, Wagner HR 2nd, et al: Zonisamide for weight loss in obese adults: a randomized controlled trial. JAMA 289:1820–1825, 2003

Goldberg JF, Burdick KE: Levetiracetam for acute mania. Am J Psychiatry 159:148, 2002

Goodwin FK, Murphy DL, Bunney WE Jr: Lithium-carbonate treatment in depression and mania: a longitudinal double-blind study. Arch Gen Psychiatry 21:486–496, 1969

Grunze H, Erfurth A, Marcuse A, et al: Tiagabine appears not to be efficacious in the treatment of acute mania. J Clin Psychiatry 60:759–762, 1999

Grunze H, Langosch J, Born C, et al: Levetiracetam in the treatment of acute mania: an open add-on study with an on-off-on design. J Clin Psychiatry 64:781–784, 2003

Hirschfeld RM, Baker JD, Wozniak P, et al: The safety and early efficacy of oral-loaded divalproex versus standard-titration divalproex, lithium, olanzapine, and placebo in the treatment of acute mania associated with bipolar disorder. J Clin Psychiatry 64:841–846, 2003a

Hirschfeld RM, Keck PE Jr, Karcher MS, et al: Rapid antimanic effect of risperidone monotherapy: a three-week, multicenter, randomized, double-blind, placebo-controlled trial. Presented at the 156th annual meeting of the American Psychiatric Association, San Francisco, CA, May 2003b

Hoopes SP, Reimherr FW, Hedges DW, et al: Treatment of bulimia nervosa with topiramate in a randomized, double-blind, placebo-controlled trial, part 1: improvement in binge and purge measures. J Clin Psychiatry 64:1335–1341, 2003

Isojarvi JI, Laatikainen TJ, Pakarinen AJ, et al: Polycystic ovaries and hyperandrogenism in women taking valproate for epilepsy. N Engl J Med 329:1383–1388, 1993

Isojarvi JI, Huuskonen UE, Pakarinen AJ, et al: The regulation of serum sodium after replacing carbamazepine with oxcarbazepine. Epilepsia 42:741–745, 2001

Jody D, McQuade RD, Carson WH Jr, et al: Efficacy of aripiprazole in subpopulations of bipolar disorder. Presented at the 157th annual meeting of the American Psychiatric Association, New York, May 2004

Joffe H, Cohen LS, Suppes T, et al: Polycystic ovarian syndrome is associated with valproate use in bipolar women. Presented at the 157th annual meeting of the American Psychiatric Association, New York, May 2004

Johnson BA, Ait-Daoud N, Bowden CL, et al: Oral topiramate for treatment of alcohol dependence: a randomised controlled trial. Lancet 361:1677–1685, 2003

Kanba S, Yagi G, Kamijima K, et al: The first open study of zonisamide, a novel anticonvulsant, shows efficacy in mania. Prog Neuropsychopharmacol Biol Psychiatry 18:707–715, 1994

Keck PE Jr, Marcus R, Tourkodimitris S, et al: A placebo-controlled, double-blind study of the efficacy and safety of aripiprazole in patients with acute bipolar mania. Am J Psychiatry 160:1651–1658, 2003a

Keck PE Jr, Versiani M, Potkin S, et al: Ziprasidone in the treatment of acute bipolar mania: a three-week, placebo-controlled, double-blind, randomized trial. Am J Psychiatry 160:741–748, 2003b

Ketter TA, Calabrese JR: Stabilization of mood from below versus above baseline in bipolar disorder: a new nomenclature. J Clin Psychiatry 63:146–151, 2002

Ketter TA, Post RM, Worthington K: Principles of clinically important drug interactions with carbamazepine, part I. J Clin Psychopharmacol 11:198–203, 1991a

Ketter TA, Post RM, Worthington K: Principles of clinically important drug interactions with carbamazepine, part II. J Clin Psychopharmacol 11:306–313, 1991b

Ketter TA, Kalali AH, Weisler RH: A 6-month, multicenter, open-label evaluation of beaded, extended-release carbamazepine capsule monotherapy in bipolar disorder patients with manic or mixed episodes. J Clin Psychiatry 65:668–673, 2004

Khanna S, Hirschfeld RMA, Karcher K, et al: Risperidone monotherapy in acute bipolar mania. Presented at the 156th annual meeting of the American Psychiatric Association, San Francisco, CA, May 2003

Kramlinger KG, Post RM: Adding lithium carbonate to carbamazepine: antimanic efficacy in treatment-resistant mania. Acta Psychiatr Scand 79:378–385, 1989

MacKinnon DF, Zandi PP, Cooper J, et al: Comorbid bipolar disorder and panic disorder in families with a high prevalence of bipolar disorder. Am J Psychiatry 159:30–35, 2002

Maggs R: Treatment of manic illness with lithium carbonate. Br J Psychiatry 109:56–65, 1963

McElroy SL, Arnold LM, Shapira NA, et al: Topiramate in the treatment of binge eating disorder associated with obesity: a randomized, placebo-controlled trial. Am J Psychiatry 160:255–261, 2003

McElroy SL, Kotwal R, Hudson JI, et al: Zonisamide in the treatment of binge-eating disorder: an open-label, prospective trial. J Clin Psychiatry 65:50–56, 2004

McIntyre RS, Mancini DA, McCann S, et al: Topiramate versus bupropion SR when added to mood stabilizer therapy for the depressive phase of bipolar disorder: a preliminary single-blind study. Bipolar Disord 4:207–213, 2002

McIntyre R, Brecher M, Paulsson B: Quetiapine as monotherapy for bipolar mania: a double-blind, randomised, parallel-group, placebo-controlled trial. Eur Neuropsychopharmacol, in press

Meehan K, Zhang F, David S, et al: A double-blind, randomized comparison of the efficacy and safety of intramuscular injections of olanzapine, lorazepam, or placebo in treating acutely agitated patients diagnosed with bipolar mania. J Clin Psychopharmacol 21:389–397, 2001

Meltzer HY, Alphs L, Green AI, et al: Clozapine treatment for suicidality in schizophrenia: International Suicide Prevention Trial (InterSePT). Arch Gen Psychiatry 60:82–91, 2003

Muller-Oerlinghausen B, Retzow A, Henn FA, et al: Valproate as an adjunct to neuroleptic medication for the treatment of acute episodes of mania: a prospective, randomized, double-blind, placebo-controlled, multicenter study. European Valproate Mania Study Group. J Clin Psychopharmacol 20:195–203, 2000

Okuma T, Yamashita I, Takahashi R, et al: Clinical efficacy of carbamazepine in affective, schizoaffective, and schizophrenic disorders. Pharmacopsychiatry 22:47–53, 1989

Pande AC, Davidson JR, Jefferson JW, et al: Treatment of social phobia with gabapentin: a placebo-controlled study. J Clin Psychopharmacol 19:341–348, 1999

Pande AC, Crockatt J, Janney CA, et al: Gabapentin Bipolar Disorder Study Group. Gabapentin in bipolar disorder: a placebo-controlled trial of adjunctive therapy. Bipolar Disord 2:249–255, 2000a

Pande AC, Pollack MH, Crockatt J, et al: Placebo-controlled study of gabapentin treatment of panic disorder. J Clin Psychopharmacol 20:467–471, 2000b

Pope HG Jr, McElroy SL, Keck PE Jr, et al: Valproate in the treatment of acute mania: a placebo-controlled study. Arch Gen Psychiatry 48:62–68, 1991

Potkin SG, Sprague R, Keck PE Jr, et al: Ziprasidone in bipolar mania: efficacy across patient subgroups. Presented at the 157th annual meeting of the American Psychiatric Association, New York, May 2004

Powers P, Sachs GS, Kushner SF, et al: Topiramate in adults with acute bipolar I mania: pooled results. Presented at the 157th annual meeting of the American Psychiatric Association, New York, May 2004

Rasgon N: The relationship between polycystic ovary syndrome and antiepileptic drugs: a review of the evidence. J Clin Psychopharmacol 24:322–334, 2004

Rattya J, Vainionpaa L, Knip M, et al: The effects of valproate, carbamazepine, and oxcarbazepine on growth and sexual maturation in girls with epilepsy. Pediatrics 103:588–593, 1999

Rosenthal M: Tiagabine for the treatment of generalized anxiety disorder: a randomized, open-label, clinical trial with paroxetine as a positive control. J Clin Psychiatry 64:1245–1249, 2003

Roth T, Walsh JK: Sleep-consolidating effects of tiagabine in patients with primary insomnia. Presented at the 157th annual meeting of the American Psychiatric Association, New York, May 2004

Rowbotham M, Harden N, Stacey B, et al: Gabapentin for the treatment of postherpetic neuralgia: a randomized controlled trial. JAMA 280:1837–1842, 1998

Sachs GS, Grossman F, Ghaemi SN, et al: Combination of a mood stabilizer with risperidone or haloperidol for treatment of acute mania: a double-blind, placebo-controlled comparison of efficacy and safety. Am J Psychiatry 159:1146–1154, 2002

Sachs G, Chengappa KN, Suppes T, et al: Quetiapine with lithium or divalproex for the treatment of bipolar mania: a randomized, double-blind, placebo-controlled study. Bipolar Disord 6:213–223, 2004a

Sachs GS, Sanchez R, Marcus RN, et al: Aripiprazole versus placebo in patients with an acute manic or mixed episode. Presented at the 157th annual meeting of the American Psychiatric Association, New York, May 2004b

Schaffer L, Schaffer C, Howe J: An open case series on the utility of tiagabine as an augmentation in refractory bipolar outpatients. J Affect Disord 71:259, 2002

Schou M, Juel-Nielsen N, Strömgren E, et al: The treatment of manic psychosis by the administration of lithium salts. J Neurol Neurosurg Psychiatry 17:250–260, 1954

Segal S, Riesenberg RA, Ice K, et al: Ziprasidone in mania: double-blind, placebo-controlled trial. Paper presented at the 56th Institute on Psychiatric Services, October 2004

Serpell MG: Gabapentin in neuropathic pain syndromes: a randomised, double-blind, placebo-controlled trial. Pain 99:557–566, 2002

Spira PJ, Beran RG: Gabapentin in the prophylaxis of chronic daily headache: a randomized, placebo-controlled study. Neurology 61:1753–1759, 2003

Stokes PE, Shamoian CA, Stoll PM, et al: Efficacy of lithium as acute treatment of manic-depressive illness. Lancet 1:1319–1325, 1971

Suppes T, Webb A, Paul B, et al: Clinical outcome in a randomized 1-year trial of clozapine versus treatment as usual for patients with treatment-resistant illness and a history of mania. Am J Psychiatry 156:1164–1169, 1999

Suppes T, Chisholm KA, Dhavale D, et al: Tiagabine in treatment refractory bipolar disorder: a clinical case series. Bipolar Disord 4:283–289, 2002

Swann AC, Bowden CL, Morris D, et al: Depression during mania: treatment response to lithium or divalproex. Arch Gen Psychiatry 54:37–42, 1997

Swann AC, Bowden CL, Calabrese JR, et al: Mania: differential effects of previous depressive and manic episodes on response to treatment. Acta Psychiatr Scand 101:444–451, 2000

Tohen M, Sanger TM, McElroy SL, et al: Olanzapine versus placebo in the treatment of acute mania: Olanzapine HGEH Study Group. Am J Psychiatry 156:702–709, 1999

Tohen M, Jacobs TG, Grundy SL, et al: Efficacy of olanzapine in acute bipolar mania: a double-blind, placebo-controlled study: the Olanzapine HGGW Study Group. Arch Gen Psychiatry 57:841–849, 2000

Tohen M, Baker RW, Altshuler LL, et al: Olanzapine versus divalproex in the treatment of acute mania. Am J Psychiatry 159:1011–1017, 2002a

Tohen M, Chengappa KN, Suppes T, et al: Efficacy of olanzapine in combination with valproate or lithium in the treatment of mania in patients partially nonresponsive to valproate or lithium monotherapy. Arch Gen Psychiatry 59:62–69, 2002b

Tohen M, Goldberg JF, Gonzalez-Pinto Arrillaga AM, et al: A 12-week, double-blind comparison of olanzapine vs haloperidol in the treatment of acute mania. Arch Gen Psychiatry 60:1218–1226, 2003

Vajda F, Lander C, O'brien T, et al: Australian pregnancy registry of women taking antiepileptic drugs. Epilepsia 45:1466, 2004

Weisler RH, Warrington L, Dunn J, et al: Adjunctive ziprasidone in bipolar mania: short-term and long-term data. Presented at the 157th annual meeting of the American Psychiatric Association, New York, May 2004a

Weisler RH, Kalali AH, Ketter TA: A multicenter, randomized, double-blind, placebo-controlled trial of extended-release carbamazepine capsules as monotherapy for bipolar disorder patients with manic or mixed episodes. J Clin Psychiatry 65:478–484, 2004b

Weisler RH, Keck PE, Swann AC, et al: Extended-release carbamazepine capsules as monotherapy for acute mania in bipolar disorder: a multicenter, randomized, double-blind, placebo-controlled trial. J Clin Psychiatry, in press

Weisler RH, Keck PE Jr, Swann AC: Treatment of manic and mixed patients with carbamazepine extended release. Presented at the 157th annual meeting of the American Psychiatric Association, New York, May, in press

Vieta E, Bourin M, Sanchez R, et al: Effectiveness of aripiprazole vs. haloperidol in the treatment of patients with acute bipolar mania over a 12-week period. Br J Psychiatry, in press

Yang Y, Nowakowska C, Becker OV, et al: Weight loss during first two months of open adjunctive zonisamide for obesity in bipolar disorder patients. Presented at the 156th annual meeting of the American Psychiatric Association, San Francisco, CA, May 2003

Yatham LN, Grossman F, Augustyns I, et al: Mood stabilisers plus risperidone or placebo in the treatment of acute mania: international, double-blind, randomised controlled trial. Br J Psychiatry 182:141–147, 2003

Yatham LN, Paulsson B, Mullen J, et al: Quetiapine versus placebo in combination with lithium or divalproex for the treatment of bipolar mania. J Clin Psychopharmacol 24:599–606, 2004

Zajecka JM, Weisler R, Sachs G, et al: A comparison of the efficacy, safety, and tolerability of divalproex sodium and olanzapine in the treatment of bipolar disorder. J Clin Psychiatry 63:1148–1155, 2002

Chapter 3

Treatment of Acute Depression in Bipolar Disorder

Gary S. Sachs, M.D.

What treatment is best for the depressed phase of bipolar disorder? This simple question can now be addressed with the help of far more pertinent study data than was available 5 years ago. Previously, even official guidelines frequently relied on tradition and extrapolation from studies that did not meet modern criteria to define evidence-based medicine. For lack of resources, discourse on the treatment of bipolar depression focused on clinical trials involving samples limited to unipolar depressed patients, a few small trials reporting results specifically for bipolar depression, and opinions derived from uncontrolled case series and clinical observation. The anemic fund of available data pertained mostly to use of what will be referred to here as "standard antidepressants," such as reuptake inhibitors, bupropion, and monoamine oxidase inhibitors (MAOIs). Beyond any guidance it provided for clinical practice, this inadequate bank of knowledge fueled two main debates about the role of standard antidepressant medications: First, are standard antidepressants efficacious for bipolar depression (even relative to their efficacy for unipolar depression)? Second, do standard antidepressant agents precipitate mania or promote cycling when given to patients with bipolar disorder?

Irrespective of their positions in these lingering debates, there is consensus among experts on the identification of bipolar depression as an area of unmet public health need (Goodwin 2003;

Hlastala et al. 1997; Silverstone and Silverstone 2004; Zornberg and Pope 1993). This chapter begins by considering bipolar depression as a public health issue and summarizing 20th century studies. After a review of recent data (limited to somatic therapies by space considerations), we will offer strategies that draw on the evidence base for practical clinical application to the management of bipolar depression.

Bipolar Depression Is an Important Public Health Problem

Episodes of bipolar depression are common and costly (Judd et al. 2003; Kupfer et al. 2002). Treatment of bipolar depression rather than mania represents the most frequent problem leading bipolar patients to enter health care systems and remains the most common clinical complaint over the entire course of illness (Judd et al. 2003; Post et al. 2003a). Although mood elevation is considered a defining feature of bipolar illness, depression tends to occur more frequently, persist longer and be associated with more disability and suicidality than episodes of abnormal mood elevation (Bottlender et al. 2000a). This widely recognized clinical need supports an aggressive approach to treatment and places treatment of bipolar depression as a top priority on the research agenda.

Consequently, while still lagging far behind unipolar depression research, the quantity and quality of data available for guiding treatment of bipolar depression has grown substantially over the past 5 years. A modest proportion of the new data sheds evidence-based light on the concerns about antidepressants and the remainder has moved the field in new directions.

Judd et al. (2002) found bipolar I patients who were followed for up to 15 years had depressive symptoms 31% of weeks versus 10% of weeks with manic, hypomanic or mixed symptoms. This 3:1 ratio of depression to mood elevation symptoms is dwarfed by the 37:1 ratio reported for bipolar II patients (52% of weeks versus 1.7% of weeks). Bryant-Comstock et al. (2002) compared privately insured bipolar patients with non-bipolar patients matched for gender and age and reported the average bipolar patient utilizes significantly more health care resources and will incur annual costs over four times greater than a non-bipolar patient ($7,663 versus $1,962). Inpatient care accounted for the biggest cost difference between groups, and was the single most costly resource in the bipolar group amounting to $2,779 compared to $398 for the non-bipolar group. Even compared to other bipolar patients with bipolar manic or mixed episodes, patients with bipolar depression incurred the highest health care costs. The increased cost associated with bipolar disorder is not due to mental health care cost alone, which accounted for only 22% of the total per-patient cost for bipolar patients and 6% of the total per-patient cost in the non-bipolar group, as the majority of the difference was related to other (non-mental health) medical care.

The high cost of care for bipolar disorder may relate to high rates of nonresponse or worsening with commonly used treatments. An analysis of clinical records for outcomes of antidepressant trials by Ghaemi et al. (2004) found nonresponse to standard antidepressants was more characteristic of bipolar depression than unipolar depression. Short-term nonresponse occurred in 51.3% of 41 patients with bipolar depression and 31.6% of 37 patients with unipolar depression. Loss of an apparent response, despite continued treatment, was 3.4 times as frequent in bipolar compared to unipolar patients, whereas withdrawal relapse into depression was 4.7 times less frequent in bipolar compared to unipolar depression. Treatment emergent affective switch (TEAS) to mania was not observed in any unipolar patient, but occurred in 84.2% of bipolar patients not taking any antimanic agent versus 31.6% taking at least one antimanic agent. Cycle acceleration and new onset rapid cycling were found only in association with bipolar depression. Newer antidepressants, in general, did not have lower rates of negative outcomes than tricyclic antidepressants.

Treatment Studies for Bipolar Depression: From the Old to the New

Thousands of articles pertaining to bipolar disorder and its treatment have been published over the past 5 years. Implicit in the process of integrating new evidence and new treatments into clinical practice is the need to weigh the available evidence, which requires a few basic concepts and a more sharply defined vocabulary. Categorizing the evidence for a treatment based on the degree to which it is supported by statistically valid inferences is essential to the process of transforming large volumes of information of unequal quality into a manageable pool of clinical knowledge. The Agency for Healthcare Research and Quality has formulated criteria for characterizing medical evidence and encourages others to adapt these criteria in authoring guidelines for local use. Many others engaged in weighing evidence use this approach in some form (American Psychiatric Association 2002; Calabrese et al. 2004b; Goodwin 2003; McIntyre et al. 2004).

The best quality evidence comes from placebo-controlled, double-blind trials in which treatment assignment is made by randomization. However, not all randomized clinical trials (RCTs) carry equal weight (for example, findings from a small, single-center study are far less compelling than those from a large multicenter study), but excessive detail regarding varieties of scientific evidence need not contribute to confusion in this chapter. Grading systems frequently employed in the construction of evidence-based guidelines can be cumbersome but are easily adapted to inform the critical analysis needed to rank treatments in routine practice. For simplicity here, the level of evidence meriting the greatest weight is termed "category A" and is used to designate evidence from studies with methodology sufficient to permit confident causal inference (e.g., placebo-controlled, randomized, double-blind study with adequate sample size or meta-analysis). This level of evidence merits an "A" rating when the trial has included an appropriate sample sufficiently large to have at least an 80% chance of detecting a difference (that is, having adequate statistical power) and provide confidence that the results are not due to chance alone.

A detailed review of statistical considerations is beyond the scope of this chapter, but three points are important to note here: First, generally accepted statistical conventions allow the interpretation of results as significantly different when the probability that the observed difference is attributable to chance alone is 5%

or less. Second, studies reporting differences insufficient to meet this standard merely fail to allow rejection of the null hypothesis and do not indicate that the conditions are the same. In other words, failure to detect a statistically significant difference does not mean treatment conditions are equivalent. This is a particular concern in studies with small sample sizes. However, if a negative study has a sufficiently large sample size, say several hundred patients, there may be sufficient statistical power to infer equivalence. Third, simple comparison of response rates for various treatments across studies can be misleading. Even sophisticated techniques which pool results from several studies (e.g., meta-analysis) are not as desirable as large single head-to-head comparisons because RCTs differ in the composition of their samples, methodology, and placebo response rates.

Effect size analysis, a serviceable but imperfect approach to comparing results from separate studies, can help attenuate the confounds of differences in placebo response rates and sample sizes. Effects size calculations are provided in several of the studies reviewed below, but even when not available, simply subtracting the placebo response rate from the response rate for the active treatment group can be a useful tool for interpreting study results.

In clinical practice, the principle of using proven treatments first requires an up-to-date knowledge of the available peer-reviewed evidence and a process of critical evaluation to weigh such data. For many decisions clinicians must confront, pertinent high-quality evidence is unavailable. Offering treatment based on the best available evidence requires assigning weight to such forms of evidence as are available. Therefore Table 3–1 provides additional criteria to help draw practical distinctions in weighing available evidence (Silverstone and Silverstone 2004), and Table 3–2 summarizes randomized controlled trials including samples with at least 60 bipolar depressed subjects.

Given the increased availability of high-quality RCT data, it is reasonable to ask the question, "Why consider naturalistic data when double blind controlled data is available?" Interpretation of open naturalistic data is indeed hazardous. Naturalistic studies can often be justified as necessary, because the very method-

Table 3–1. Category of evidence for widely used psychotropics

Medication (best citation)	Evidence of efficacy for bipolar depression
Olanzapine + fluoxetine (Tohen et al. 2003)	A
Lamotrigine (Calabrese et al. 1999)	A
Quetiapine (Calabrese et al. 2004a)	A
Olanzapine (Tohen et al. 2003)	A
Standard antidepressants (Gijsman et al. 2004)[a]	B
Imipramine (Cohn et al. 1989)	B
Desipramine (Sachs et al. 1994)[b]	C
Imipramine (Nemeroff et al. 2001)	F
Fluoxetine (Cohn et al. 1989)	B
Paroxetine (Nemeroff et al. 2001)[c]	B
Sertraline (Post et al. 2003a)	B
Citalopram (Kupfer et al. 2001)	C
Bupropion (Sachs et al. 1994)	B
Tranylcypromine (Himmelhoch et al. 1991)	B
Selegiline (Mendlewicz and Youdim 1980)	B
Moclobemide (Silverstone 2001)	B
Pramipexole (Goldberg et al. 2004)	B
Lithium (Nemeroff et al. 2001)	B
Divalproex (Davis et al., in press)	B
Carbamazepine (Post et al. 1986)	D
Gabapentin (Frye et al. 2000)	D
Topiramate (Vieta et al. 2002)	D
Oxcarbazepine	E-
Aripiprazole (Worthington et al. 2005)	D
Clozapine	E
Haloperidol	E-

Table 3–1. Category of evidence for widely used psychotropics *(continued)*

Medication (best citation)	Evidence of efficacy for bipolar depression
Risperidone (Ostroff and Nelson 1999)	D
Ziprasidone	E-
Omega-3 (Post et al. 2003a)	F

Category
A: Double-blind, placebo controlled trials with adequate sample size
B: Double-blind, controlled trials without placebo or not completely satisfying the requirements above
C: Open trials can be very valuable when controlled and are most informative when the treatments being compared are assigned by randomization. Such trials can be categorized as C and C+, respectively
D: Uncontrolled observations, case series and even single case reports can provide a rationale for selecting treatment and can be categorized D and D–, respectively
E: In the absence of published studies, treatments can be rated E+ or E– depending on whether or not category A evidence supports a class effect treatment
F: Controlled trials with negative result
[a]Meta-analysis suggests a class effect; [b]No difference from bupropion in a small comparator study; [c]Superior to placebo adjunct in post hoc analysis restricted to subjects with Li<0.8 mmol

ologies of randomization and blinding that give a controlled trial scientific rigor can limit the generalizability of RCT results to the broader population actually seeking treatment. This may account for a part of the efficacy-effectiveness gap: the difference between the results obtained in clinical trials versus open clinical practice.

The extent to which RCT results are influenced by who enters the study (accession bias) limits their applicability to real-world practice. Many, if not most, typical clinic patients would be excluded by eligibility criteria commonly employed in RCT studies. Some eligible subjects may be unwilling to accept the limited treatment options available within a randomized study. Naturalistic effectiveness reports are, therefore, of great interest particu-

Table 3–2. Acute trials reporting results for bipolar depression (*n*=60)

Authors	Active agents	Response rate[a] Active	Response rate[a] Control	Duration
Calabrese	Lamotrigine 50 mg	48%	Placebo 29%	7 weeks
	Lamotrigine 200 mg	54%		
Tohen	Olanzapine	33%	Placebo 25%	8 weeks
	Olanzapine+fluoxetine	49%		
Calabrese	Quetiapine 300 mg	58%	Placebo 22%	8 weeks
	Quetiapine 600 mg	58%		
Nemeroff	Lithium+paroxetine	46%	Lithium +	10 weeks
	Lithium+imipramine	39%	Placebo 35%	
Silverstone	Moclobemide±MS	46%	Imipramine ±MS 53%	8 weeks
Vieta	Venalfaxine±MS	48%	Paroxetine ±MS 43%	6 weeks

Note. MS=lithium or valproate.
[a] Response rate defined as percentage with 50% improvement on MADRS or Ham-D.

larly when formal prospective outcome assessments are reported. Use of rating scales in naturalistic studies not only allows an assessment of treatment under conditions more generalizable to routine clinical practice but also permits quantitative comparison with the results obtained in RCTs. When similar results are obtained from RCTs and naturalistic studies, firm conclusions can be drawn. Dissimilar results require explanation. Poor outcome in a naturalistic study is of concern, particularly in the absence of more encouraging controlled data.

Vocabulary Problems

Clinical use of imprecise terms frequently plagues psychiatry. The utility of terms such as "mood stabilizer" and "antidepressant" are compromised by the variety of meanings attached to them by the general public as well as by psychiatrists.

The "mood stabilizer" concept originated as a term to convey the bimodal activity of lithium in recognition of its antidepressant as well as antimanic effects. The term is now often applied to merely designate medications marketed for bipolar disorder without any precise meaning. This is problematic, because there is no consensus definition of "mood stabilizer" and no regulatory authority has actually approved any treatment as a "mood stabilizer." One unfortunate consequence of the term "mood stabilizer" is the perception that experts recommend withholding "antidepressants" from bipolar patients diagnosed with depression. Recommendations suggesting use of a "mood stabilizer" as initial treatment for bipolar depression leaves many patients confused and strains the therapeutic alliance. In this chapter the term "mood stabilizer" will refer to lithium, valproate, and carbamazepine and will be used sparingly in instances where other terms might introduce even worse confusion. In order to preserve the possibility of classifying all agents proven efficacious against depression as "antidepressants," agents approved for treatment of unipolar depression will be referred to as "standard antidepressants."

The terms "antidepressant-induced mania" or "antidepressant-induced affective switch" will be avoided entirely since they imply a causal role in phenomena they can only describe. Instead, "treatment emergent affective switch" (TEAS) will be used as a cause neutral term indicating a change from depression or mania to a pathological mood state of the opposite polarity.

A Brief Review of 20th-Century Studies

Standard antidepressant medications such as reuptake inhibitors, bupropion, and MAOIs added to lithium, valproate, or carbamazepine have long been and remain the most widely prescribed treatments for bipolar depression. Surprisingly few randomized controlled studies of standard antidepressants have been carried out with adequately sized samples of depressed bipolar patients. Relatively small double-blind studies conducted in the 20th century investigated the use of adjunctive imipramine, bupropion, desipramine, fluoxetine, moclobemide, and tranylcypromine for bipolar depression and have been reviewed previously (Calabrese et al. 1999; Zornberg and Pope 1993). Until recently, these randomized controlled clinical trials represented the best available data supporting the use of standard antidepressants for bipolar disorder; all lacked adequate statistical power, many allowed inconsistent use of concomitant mood stabilizers, and several used comparators other than placebo. Beyond these limitations, variations in study duration and response criteria make it hazardous to compare results across studies. For example, most studies define response as 50% improvement from the baseline depression rating scale score, but there is no systematic method for correction of improved depression scores that occur concurrently with TEAS to mania. About a quarter of the impressive response rates reported in some studies of tranylcypromine and imipramine monotherapy represent subjects who became manic during the study (Himmelhoch et al. 1991). Although no 20th century study of standard antidepressants meets category A criteria, this body of data has established benchmarks against which treatments for bipolar depression can be measured.

The most rigorous of the 20th century controlled studies of standard antidepressants compared placebo, imipramine, and paroxetine as adjuncts to lithium for treatment of bipolar depression. Initially presented in 1997 and published by Nemeroff et al. in 2001, this double-blind, controlled trial randomized 117 depressed bipolar patients treated with lithium (serum $Li \geq 0.5$ mmol/L) to add paroxetine ($n=35$), imipramine ($n=39$), or placebo ($n=43$) for 10 weeks. Therapeutic response was defined as having a final Hamilton Rating Scale for Depression (Ham-D) score ≤ 7 or Clinical Global Impression (CGI) Scale of improvement score ≤ 2 (at least moderate improvement). Overall response rates for those receiving adjunctive paroxetine, imipramine, or placebo (Ham-D criterion: 45.5%, 38.9%, and 34.9%, respectively; CGI criterion: 54.5%, 58.3%, and 46.5% respectively) were not significantly different. A post hoc analysis limited to those subjects with serum lithium levels ≤ 0.8 mmol/L, however, did find significantly greater improvement in both the paroxetine+lithium and the imipramine+lithium group compared to the placebo+lithium group (Ham-D criterion: 52.6%, 36.8%, and 31.8%, respectively; CGI criterion: 52.6%, 68.4%, and 40.9%, respectively). This study did not use a formal scale to assess manic symptoms, and not surprisingly reported low rates of treatment emergent mania. Paroxetine did not precipitate a full manic episode in any patient, but 7.7% of patients receiving imipramine and 2.3% of patients in the placebo group did meet criteria for mania. While the reported frequency of full manic episodes was low, these and similarly reassuring data reported by other studies should be viewed in the ethical context of a RCT, in which signs of impending mania would preclude continuation of antidepressant treatment under double-blind conditions. Patients presenting with significant evidence of abnormal mood elevation subthreshold for mania are typically removed from the study and reported as an adverse event, "manic reaction," but not as an episode of mania or hypomania. Important limitations of this study include the absence of reporting baseline or changes in mania rating scale scores.

Kupfer and colleagues reported results from an 8-week open, acute study with an interesting design variation. The antidepressant efficacy of citalopram was evaluated as an adjunct to treatment with lithium, valproate, or carbamazepine±antipsychotics ±hypnotics/anxiolytics in a multicenter trial that permitted enrollment of bipolar I and bipolar II subjects, but lacked both randomization and blinding (Kupfer et al. 2001). The formal assessment methodology typical of controlled efficacy trials was used to collect depression and mania ratings prospectively. The open design intended to capitalize on removing what are generally regarded as major barriers to enrollment in multicenter intervention studies: the use of placebo and the need to accept randomization. The study design also anticipated a higher response rate than might be expected in a blinded trial. Surprisingly, not only did the study fall far short of its recruitment target, but only 21 of the 45 (47%) enrolled subjects met the acute response criteria (50% improvement from baseline Ham-D score at week 8). Follow-up for an additional 16 weeks revealed that 14 patients (31.1%) achieved a sustained remission. In view of the limitations of uncontrolled open data, this outcome might best serve as a standard for comparison with other studies. Important limitations of this study include the absence of reporting TEAS or changes in Young Mania Rating Scale (YMRS) scores.

While bipolar I patients are routinely excluded from monotherapy trials testing standard antidepressants, bipolar II subjects are often eligible. Amsterdam extracted results for bipolar II subjects participating in two double-blind studies (Amsterdam 1998). The first, a 6-week trial compared venlafaxine (up to 225 mg) administered on single versus multiple daily dosing schedules. The Ham-D and the Montgomery-Åsberg Depression Rating Scale (MADRS) were used to rate depressive symptoms. There was no difference in response to single versus split dosing. Bipolar II subjects ($n=17$) appeared to respond earlier than unipolar depressives ($n=31$), and no TEAS was observed in either group. In the second study, bipolar II and unipolar patients enrolled in a double-blind fluoxetine trial were found to respond to similarly, and TEAS was observed in 3.8% of the bipolar group and none of the unipolar group (Amsterdam et al. 1998). The same investigator recently reported results extracted from the open treatment phase of a study intending to randomize fluoxetine responders to a double-blind maintenance study (Amsterdam et al. 2004). The sample included 37 depressed bipolar II subjects who received 20 mg of fluoxetine and were followed with formal rating scales for mania as well as depression. Of the bipolar subjects, 38% met response criteria, 7.3% had symptoms suggestive of hypomania, and one patient stopped treatment due to "a rapid mood swing into depression." Important limitations of these studies include the absence of reporting baseline or changes in mania rating scale scores.

Lithium

The 2002 edition of the *American Psychiatric Association Practice Guideline for the Treatment of Patients With Bipolar Disorder* recommends lithium as an initial treatment for bipolar depression of mild to moderate severity. Based on observations in his initial case series in the late 1940s which included three chronically depressed patients who did not improve following administration of lithium, Cade (1949) concluded lithium did not have antidepressant effects. However, several small controlled trials conducted between 1968 and 1976 indicated lithium has an antidepressant benefit. Authors of several early reports acknowledged finding that lithium indeed had antidepressant efficacy, but qualified it as being less robust or having slower onset than standard antidepressants (Dunner et al. 1976; Fieve et al. 1968). There remains little statistical evidence by which to compare the efficacy of lithium relative to standard antidepressants. The best data addressing this issue directly comes from a post hoc analysis in the aforementioned double-blind, controlled trial in which Nemeroff et al. (2001) found no overall benefit from adding a standard antidepressant compared to adding placebo to lithium. In the subgroup of patients with serum lithium levels above 0.8 mEq/L, a trend was found indicating better outcome in the lithium plus placebo group compared to lithium plus either of the standard antidepressants, but did not reach statistical significance. Notably, this study enrolled bipolar subjects who met criteria for major depression and were often already receiving lithium treatment without benefit at the time of study entry. The study results, therefore, likely understate the antidepressant efficacy of lithium due to the enrollment of subjects who demonstrated nonresponse to lithium prior to intake.

Lamotrigine

In 1999, results of the first category A bipolar depression study, a 7-week, parallel group, double-blind RCT, were published which found both 50 mg and 200 mg of lamotrigine were superior to placebo for treatment of depression in bipolar subjects (N=195) (Calabrese et al. 1999). Criteria for response and 50% improvement from baseline MADRS score was met by 29%, 48%, and 54% of subjects in the placebo, lamotrigine 50 mg, and lamotrigine 200 mg groups respectively. This study also used a formal mania rating scale (first 11 items from the Schedule for Affective Disorders and Schizophrenia—Change Version [SAD-C MRS]) to evaluate TEAS into mania. There were no significant differences between the groups at any time point on mean SAD-C MRS scores. Furthermore, rates of TEAS reported qualitatively as adverse effects were low (lamotrigine 5.4% versus placebo 4.6%) and did not differ between the treatment groups. Headache was the only adverse effect that occurred significantly more often in the active treatment groups (32% to 35%) compared to placebo (17%). Overall rates of rash (11% to 14%) and discontinuation due to rash (3% to 6%) were similar across groups, and no serious rash was reported in any group.

Update: 21st-Century Studies

Category A Studies

Already, research in the 21st century has brought a substantial increase in both the quantity and quality of studies. Several category A studies have been completed, however few controlled trials conducted after 2000 report results for standard antidepressants. This includes a study evaluating the selective serotonin reuptake inhibitor, fluoxetine in combination with olanzapine, and two rigorous double-blind, controlled comparisons of various standard antidepressants. In addition, category A data are available for monotherapy use of olanzapine and quetiapine.

In the largest placebo-controlled, double-blind trial yet published for bipolar depression, Tohen and colleagues randomized 833 bipolar I subjects meeting criteria for a major depressive episode. This study found a slight but statistically significant advantage for olanzapine (n=370) over placebo (n=377) and a robust statistically significant advantage for the combination of olanzapine and fluoxetine over olanzapine (n=86) and placebo (Tohen et al. 2003). Response was achieved by significantly more subjects receiving combined treatment (48.8%) than those receiving olanzapine (32.8%) or placebo (24.5%). The advantage of active treatments over placebo reached statistical significance at the week 1 assessment and effect size analysis revealed a small effect for olanzapine (0.32) and a moderate effect for the combination of olanzapine and fluoxetine (0.68) (Calabrese et al. 2004a). The addition of fluoxetine did not offset the weight gain or sedation associated with olanzapine. The FDA has approved the combination of olanzapine and fluoxetine for treatment of bipolar depression.

Even the modest antidepressant efficacy demonstrated for olanzapine monotherapy in bipolar I depressed subjects must be regarded as the beginning of an evidence base regarding the utility of a new therapeutic class agent for bipolar depression, namely the atypical antipsychotics.

Recently Calabrese et al. (2004a) presented results from a large category A, double-blind trial that randomized 542 depressed bipolar I and bipolar II subjects to placebo, quetiapine 300 mg, or quetiapine 600 mg. Overall 300 mg and 600 mg doses of quetiapine both produced significantly higher responder rates (both 58%) at 8 weeks than placebo (36%). Separation from placebo was evident by week 1. Both doses of quetiapine demonstrated a statistically significant advantage over placebo on change from baseline MADRS and were associated with moderate effect sizes (0.64 and 0.75, respectively). Subgroup analyses revealed the effect size to be small in bipolar II subjects and large in bipolar I subjects. On each of the 10 individual MADRS items including suicidal ideation, statistically significant differences were obtained favoring active treatment. Dry mouth, sedation, and hypotension were the most commonly reported adverse effects. Discontinuation for any adverse event was seen in 8.3% of patients on placebo, 16.2% with quetiapine 300 mg, and 26.1% with quetiapine 600 mg.

Category B Studies: Randomized Comparator Studies Without Placebo Control

There have been several noteworthy recent category B studies, one of these involved moclobemide, a reversible inhibitor of MAO type A that is not approved in the United States but approved in Canada as well as multiple European and South American countries for treatment of depression. In a randomized, double-blind, parallel group, multicenter study with the largest sample receiving standard antidepressants for bipolar depression, Silverstone and colleagues (2001) compared moclobemide 450–750 mg/day ($n=81$) and imipramine 150–250 mg/day ($n=75$). Lithium and/or an anticonvulsant mood stabilizer were used concomitantly by 59.4% in the moclobemide group and 64.0% of imipramine-treated subjects. Outcome was assessed using the 17-item Ham-D, the MADRS, and the YMRS. Although no statistically significant differences were found between the two groups on any efficacy measure, trends favored imipramine over moclobemide on both change from baseline Ham-D scores (13.0 versus 9.9) and change from baseline MADRS scores (17.6 versus 13.2). Furthermore, the proportion meeting the remission criteria (total Ham-D score of at least 50% and/or final score of 10 or less) was 46% in the moclobemide group and 53% in the imipramine group. Withdrawal from the study due to treatment emergent mania occurred in 3.7% of patients on moclobemide and 11% on imipramine, but the difference was not statistically significant. Treatment emergent mood elevation was generally more severe in the imipramine group, with 6.7% having a YMRS score of 18 or more compared to 2.5% on moclobemide. Anticholinergic side effects and weight gain were significantly more common with imipramine than moclobemide.

The Stanley Foundation Bipolar Network (SFBN) reported preliminary results of a double-blind comparison in which bupropion (up to 450 mg/day), sertraline (up to 200 mg/day), or venlafaxine (up to 375 mg/day) was added to ongoing "mood stabilizer" treatment (Post 2001). Subjects included 64 bipolar patients who participated in 95 randomized acute treatment phases at five sites in a 10-week, double-blind trial for depression and a 1-year blinded continuation maintenance phase for responders. Improvement on the Clinical Global Impression Scale for Bipolar Disorder (CGI-BP) and the occurrence of hypomania or mania was determined by review of daily ratings on the National Institute of Mental Health–Life Chart Methodology. Overall, 37% of 95 acute treatment phases in which antidepressant treatment was used as an adjunct to mood stabilizers were associated with a much or very much improved rating on the CGI-BP for depression and 14% were associated with TEAS to mood elevation. Among the 48 who responded and entered continuation phase treatment, one-third also experienced TEAS.

While the above comparison of sertraline, bupropion, or venlafaxine remained blinded, updated results for affective switch have been presented with an enlarged sample of 127 bipolar depressed patients. Data was available for a total of 175 acute antidepressant augmentation trials because nonresponders were re-randomized. Overall 9.1% of the acute trials were associated with switches into clinically significant hypomania or mania (with at least moderate symptom intensity) and another 9.1% with a week or more of milder hypomania (with no to minimal dysfunction). Acute treatment responders were offered a year of continuation treatment and 73 agreed to participate. Of these continuation phase antidepressant trials, 35.6% were associated with affective switch (16.4% hypomanic to manic and 19.2% hypomanic).

Vieta and colleagues carried out a 6-week, randomized, single-blind comparison in which paroxetine (n=30) or venlafaxine (n=30) was added to ongoing treatment with lithium, valproate, carbamazepine, or other putative mood stabilizers (Vieta et al. 2002). Intention-to-treat analysis revealed no significant efficacy differences between the treatments, with 43% (n=13) of patients taking paroxetine and 47% (n=14) taking venlafaxine meeting criteria for treatment response. The rate of TEAS was only 3% (n=1) in the paroxetine group, but 13% (n=4) in the venlafaxine group.

Bipolar patients frequently experience so-called breakthrough depressive episodes, which are recurrences despite ongoing treatment with a mood stabilizer. Two small studies have specifically addressed the issue of whether it is more desirable to add a standard antidepressant or a second presumptive mood stabilizer.

Young and colleagues randomized 27 subjects who became depressed during ongoing treatment with lithium or valproate to adjunctive treatment with paroxetine or the combination of lithium and valproate for 6 weeks (Young et al. 2000). Ham-D scores improved similarly in both groups, but there were significantly more dropouts due to adverse events in the lithium plus valproate treatment group than in the group treated with paroxetine plus lithium or valproate.

McIntyre et al. (2002) used blinded raters to compare the efficacy and tolerability of topiramate, an anticonvulsant reported to have antimanic properties in uncontrolled observations but, as described in Chapter 2, failed to demonstrate efficacy as monotherapy for mania in adults, and sustained release bupropion (bupropion SR) added to ongoing mood stabilizer therapy in 36 depressed bipolar out-patients. At baseline, these mood stabilizer treated subjects had Ham-D-17 scores ≥ 16 and were randomized to receive adjunctive treatment consisting of escalating dosages of either topiramate (50–300 mg/day) or bupropion SR (100–400 mg/day) for 8 weeks. Nearly the same percentage of patients in the topiramate group (56%) and the bupropion SR group (59%) experienced a 50% improvement from baseline. Both topiramate and bupropion SR were generally well tolerated and no cases of TEAS were observed. Mean weight loss was greater in the topiramate group (5.8 kg) than the bupropion SR group (1.2 kg).

These preliminary data do not suffice to support any definite conclusions, particularly with respect to comparative efficacy. Small studies without placebo control groups showing equivalent active comparator results could indicate that the treatments were equally effective, equally ineffective, or simply that the study lacked sensitivity or statistical power to detect any actual differences. In addition, although the significant findings with respect to tolerability and weight effects are of interest, they need to be replicated with larger samples.

Category C Studies: Naturalistic Comparison Studies Without Randomization

Several other reports have been published pertinent to the use of standard antidepressants, which did not involve randomization. When considering findings from these studies, several caveats should be kept in mind: uncontrolled data is notoriously unreliable. Even when results for comparison groups are included to create a quasi-experimental study, naturalistic results must be interpreted with great caution as naturalistic studies are subject to many forms of unmeasured bias. The confounding influence of such biases are mitigated in RCTs by virtue of random assignment which can create balanced comparison groups, while non-randomized studies lack this compensatory mechanism. For instance, results from open studies that use prospective ratings are subject to bias which might influence outcome such as differential expectation of adverse effects or efficacy. When clinicians recommend the treatment they believe is the most potent for patients perceived as more severely ill or having less likelihood of response, that treatment would likely be disadvantaged relative to those considered for mildly ill or more responsive patients. Furthermore, enthusiasm for a treatment studied under open conditions may account for the high rates of response typically observed in early uncontrolled observations. Conversely, entrance into double-blind, placebo-controlled trials may be most acceptable for patients with mild to moderate severity and lead to results which do not generalize to broader clinical populations. With these caveats in mind, however, naturalistic results can still be illuminating.

Altshuler and colleagues reported naturalistic outcomes for 1,078 subjects treated at SFBN sites. About half ($n=549$) of this sample became depressed and had a standard antidepressant medication added to their ongoing treatment regimen for at least 1 day and 189 patients continued antidepressant treatment at least 60 days. Only 84 patients met study criteria for remission of 6 consecutive weeks with a Clinical Global Impression for Severity of Illness (CGI-S) score ≤ 2 (current symptoms of depression were too few or too mild to clearly indicate presence of illness) (Altshuler et al. 2003). This requirement for a durable remission is much more clinically meaningful than the response criteria used in typical efficacy studies. The responders represent only 15% of those for whom there was a clinical intent to treat with standard antidepressant medication. Among subjects who met the 6-week remission criteria, comparison groups were constructed retrospectively based on whether antidepressants were continued following the recovery for more than 6 months or discontinued before 6 months. The study did not attempt to control or influence the clinician's choice about when to discontinue antidepressant treatment. Over the first 4 months, about 20–25% experienced a relapse into depression regardless of whether antidepressants were continued or not. A significantly lower rate of relapse into depression over 1 year was, however, observed for those who remained on antidepressants (36%), compared with those who discontinued antidepressant medications during the first 6 months (70%). For subjects whose clinicians chose to continue antidepressants, there was no increase in the rate of TEAS compared with subjects whose clinician chose to stop antidepressants. Interpretation of this outcome may be confounded, in part, by a lack of knowledge of why or exactly when clinicians decided to continue or discontinue antidepressant medication. If a patient relapsed in month 2 despite continued antidepressant treatment and the clinician decided to discontinue ineffective treatment, their assignment to the less-than-6-months group would be a consequence of poor outcome rather than a cause. Nevertheless, these results suggest no reason to routinely discontinue sustained successful antidepressant therapy since the risk associated with standard antidepressants appears to be largely in the first 2–6 months of treatment.

Sachs (2003a) reported preliminary outcomes for the first 1,000 subjects enrolled in the National Institute of Mental Health (NIMH)–sponsored Systematic Treatment Enhancement Program for Bipolar Disorder (STEP-BD). During the first year of follow-up, 181 subjects experienced the new onset of at least one episode meeting criteria for major depression, including 50 who experienced multiple depressive episodes. STEP-BD uses a standardized clinical monitoring form to collect prospective assessments of symptom severity and assigns a clinical status based on DSM-IV-TR criteria at every follow-up visit (Sachs 2004; Sachs et al. 2003). Analysis of treatment outcome for the first episode of depression revealed no statistically significant advantage for adding standard antidepressant medication. In fact, the trend indicated a shorter time to mee DSM-IV-TR criteria for "recovered," defined as 8 consecutive weeks euthymic (no more than two moderate symptoms) for the group receiving treatment with neither a standard antidepressant nor lamotrigine (100 days), compared to those receiving a standard antidepressant without lamotrigine (118 days, $P<0.08$), those receiving a standard antidepressant with lamotrigine (136 days, $P<0.15$), and those receiving lamotrigine without a standard antidepressant (163 days, $P<0.46$). Surprisingly the rates of TEAS were 14.6% in both the group managed with neither a standard antidepressant nor lamotrigine and those managed with both. Lower TEAS rates were observed in subjects receiving a standard antidepressant (8.6% of 152) or lamotrigine (8.8% of 41). These marginally significant results indicate that the best efficacy and worst TEAS rates were associated with the clinical intent to manage without adding standard antidepressants. While baseline severity ratings for depression and mania were similar, the groups differed at baseline on other clinical dimensions such as number of prior episodes, history of TEAS, and bipolar subtype. Thus, like the results above from Altshuler, nonrandomized, quasi-experimental data must be interpreted cautiously. The clinicians managing these patients may often select treatment based on a prognostic estimate; those thought most likely to respond and those thought most likely to experience TEAS receive the treatment perceived as most benign.

In a separate examination of data from STEP-BD, Truman et al. (2004) found 19.5% of 1,250 retrospectively reported antidepressant trials were associated with affective switch within the first 12 weeks of treatment. While this report did not establish causality, subjects reporting a history of TEAS were found to have a significantly higher conditional probability of subsequent treatment emergent switches, particularly if they were reexposed to antidepressants of the same class as that associated with an index episode of TEAS.

Summary of Standard Antidepressants

The role of standard antidepressants in the treatment of bipolar depression remains a matter of considerable controversy. While no single medication has regulatory approval specifically for bipolar depression (to date, only the combination of fluoxetine with olanzapine has such approval), the preponderance of evidence available from a handful of small studies is consistent with the notion that medications effective for treatment of unipolar

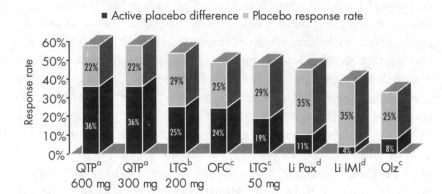

Figure 3–1. Treatment response in modern trials with >100 depressed bipolar subjects.

Each bar represents the response rate for an active treatment and is divided into segments indicating the placebo response rate in the trial and the difference between active and placebo response in that trial.

Note. IMI = imipramine; LTG = lamotrigine; Li = lithium; OFC= olanzapine + flouxetine combination; Olz = olanzapine; Pax = paroxetine; QTP = quetiapine [a]Calabrese et al. 2004; [b]Calabrese et al. 1999; [c]Tohen et al. 2003; [d]Nemeroff et al. 2001

depression may be more effective than placebo for the treatment of bipolar depression (Gijsman et al. 2004). Figure 3–1 compares the response rate for active treatments at their endpoints and the magnitude of difference between response to the active agents and placebo comparators in modern trials with samples greater than 80 subjects. The benefit of adding standard antidepressant medications or olanzapine appears modest compared to lamotrigine, quetiapine, or olanzapine combined with fluoxetine, but such comparisons (aside from olanzapine plus fluoxetine compared to olanzapine monotherapy) lack the validity of an RCT making a direct head-to-head comparison. Finally, some evidence supports the contention that at least a small subgroup of patients with bipolar disorder who respond well to adjunctive antidepressants for a few months may have better long-term outcomes when these antidepressants are continued rather than discontinued.

While the causal link between antidepressant and TEAS is not well established, the risk of TEAS can be quantified. The rates of TEAS observed prospectively in the SFBN and STEP-BD suggest 8–15% of depressed bipolar subjects will have clinically significant TEAS over the first 3 months of antidepressant treatment. Meta-analysis of controlled trials suggests the risk of TEAS associated with tricyclic antidepressants is about threefold higher than TEAS risk associated with other classes of antidepressants (Gijsman et al. 2004). It appears likely that the risk of TEAS is substantially higher in subjects reporting prior TEAS, particularly if they are rechallenged with an agent that yielded TEAS or an agent from the same class of antidepressant that resulted in TEAS.

Valproate and Related Compounds

As with Cade's unenthusiastic assessment of lithium as a treatment for depression, Lambert's report of an uncontrolled cases series suggested valpromide had little antidepressant effect (Lambert and Venaud 1987; Lambert et al. 1966) and may have unduly shaped perception of the psychotropic properties of valpromide and related compounds. It is likely, however, that much of the sample Lambert referred to as manic-depressive consisted of patients who would today be considered as having recurrent unipolar depression.

One group found that in 19 mood stabilizer-naïve, depressed, bipolar II disorder patients, open divalproex monotherapy, with a mean dosage of 882 mg/day and serum concentration of 81 µg/mL, yielded a 63% overall response rate; 11 medication-naïve patients tended to have a higher response rate compared to eight patients with prior exposure to stimulants or antidepressants (82% versus 38%) (Winsberg et al. 2001). This finding prompted small, randomized, placebo-controlled, double-blind pilot studies. One such study in bipolar I and bipolar II disorder patients with acute bipolar depression reported that patients on divalproex ($n=21$, mean maximum dosage 1,391 mg/day) tended to improve more than those on placebo ($n=22$) at some time points, but failed to separate from placebo, perhaps due to the limited sample size or suboptimal (62 µg/mL) blood valproate concentrations (Sachs et al. 2001). Another such study reported statistically significant antidepressant effect for divalproex ($n=13$) compared to placebo ($n=12$) in an 8-week, double-blind study (Davis et al., in press). Ham-D scores improved by 43.5% in the active treatment group and 27.0% in the placebo treated group. Mean serum valproate levels were 80 ± 9.3 μg/mL at week 4 and 81 ± 19.2 μg/mL at week 8.

Spontaneous, adverse effects were unremarkable in these studies, however, gastrointestinal complaints and weight gain are common among valproate treated patients. Use of valproate is limited by concerns about several adverse effects (hepatotoxicity, pancreatitis, teratogenicity). Enzyme inhibition is common with valproate and can double the half-life of some drugs, such as lamotrigine. Among premenopausal bipolar women, Joffe and colleagues found valproate use was associated with a 10% incidence of treatment emergent polycystic ovarian syndrome (Joffe et al. 2004).

Carbamazepine

Antidepressant effects of carbamazepine have been reported in two small randomized, double-blind studies that used cross-over design (Ballenger and Post 1980; Post et al. 1986). In the larger of these studies, 35 depressed patients diagnosed by DSM-III criteria participated in a double-blind study of the acute antidepressant effects of the anticonvulsant carbamazepine, and 12 (34.3%) showed more than mild improvement. The average carbamazepine dosage was 971 mg/day with a mean serum concentration of 9.3 ± 1.9 mg/mL.

Joffe et al. (1987) considered whether the improvement seen in depression ratings might be secondary to nonspecific sedation effects. Motor activity in 19 depressed patients treated with carbamazepine was measured using wrist activity monitors. Improvement in depression was associated with significant increases in motor activity but motor activity in nonresponders was not decreased. Thus the benefit of carbamazepine did not appear to be merely due to sedative effects.

Use of carbamazepine is limited by the concern over several adverse effects (aplastic anemia, rash, hyponatremia, hepatotoxicity, memory impairment, teratogenicity) and drug–drug interactions, which are particularly problematic given the high rates of polypharmacy and use of oral contraceptives in clinical populations. Enzyme induction is common with carbamazepine and does not appear limited to cytochrome 3A4. In addition to reduction of carbamazepine serum levels, enzyme induction leads to increased metabolism of diverse categories of medication, including antipsychotics, antidepressants, anticonvulsants, and oral contraceptives.

Electroconvulsive Therapy

Treatment guidelines often recommend electroconvulsive therapy (ECT) as an evidence-based option for bipolar depression despite the absence of category A evidence (American Psychiatric Association 2002; Goodwin 2003; Royal Australian and New Zealand College of Psychiatrists Clinical Practice Guidelines Team for Deliberate Self-Harm 2004). However, controlled studies of ECT for major depression have shown ECT to be highly efficacious and obtain similar positive results for subgroups of bipolar subjects as well as unipolar subjects. Further support for ECT comes from case series that describe beneficial results for bipolar patients refractory to conventional antidepressant medication (Prudic et al. 1990). Daly and colleagues studied differences in response to electroconvulsive therapy between patients with bipolar ($n=66$) or unipolar ($n=162$) major depression over three double-blind treatment protocols. Symptomatic change on Ham-D scores evaluated by a blinded evaluation team revealed no difference in rates of response or remission following the ECT course, or in response to unilateral or bilateral ECT. In comparison to unipolar subjects, both bipolar I and bipolar II patients showed more rapid response to ECT and received significantly fewer ECT treatments than unipolar patients (Daly et al. 2001). As might be expected, however, lower response rates are observed in routine clinical practice. In contrast to the 70%–90% remission rates expected with ECT in study reports (Black et al. 1986), Prudic et al. found less impressive remission rates (30.3%–46.7%) in a community sample (Prudic et al. 2004).

Novel Therapeutics: The Search for More Efficacious Treatments

Adjunctive Stimulants

Given the important role of dopamine in reward and initiation of motivated behavior, the use of dopamine agonists appears as an attractive option for treatment of bipolar depression, but not until the 21st century has even scant RCT data become available. Stimulants have long been reported beneficial based on case series but have also been associated with worsening mania, irritability, or psychosis (Cassano et al. 2004; El-Mallakh 2000; Murphy et al. 1973; Perugi et al. 2001; Shopsin and Gershon 1978). In considering the role of stimulants it is prudent to keep in mind that several of these reports describe early positive results that were lost with continued treatment.

Consistent with these findings, El-Mallakh (2000) published results of an open, uncontrolled case series in which methylphenidate was added to ongoing mood stabilizer treatment for bipolar depression ($n=15$). Mean MADRS improved from 16.9 ± 1.79 at baseline to 9.4 ± 9.73 on week 12 ($P=0.12$) and 20% dropped out due to anxiety, agitation, and hypomania.

Adjunctive Dopamine Receptor Agonists

Promising open results suggesting that the dopamine receptor agonist pramipexole possesses antidepressant properties have been tested in two very small single-center, placebo-controlled, double-blind studies. Goldberg and colleagues randomized treatment-resistant, nonpsychotic, depressed outpatients with bipolar I or bipolar II disorder to 6 weeks of treatment with pramipexole ($n=12$) or placebo ($n=10$) added to existing therapy with lithium, divalproex, carbamazepine, lamotrigine, and/or gabapentin at stable dosages for one month, and lorazepam (up to 2 mg/day) or clonazepam (up to 1 mg/day) were permitted as needed for insomnia or agitation (Goldberg et al. 2004). Administration of blinded pramipexole was started at 0.125 mg twice daily and increased by 0.25 mg/day every 3–5 days to a target range of 1.0–2.5 mg/day. For subjects unresponsive at the target dosage, further increases continued up to 5.0 mg/day, with a mean final dosage of 1.7 mg/day. Significantly more pramipexole-treated subjects (67% of 12) than placebo-treated subjects (20% of 10) improved by at least 50% from their baseline Ham-D scores. Only one patient dropped out due to adverse events (due to psychotic mania while taking pramipexole).

Zarate and colleagues undertook a double-blind, placebo-controlled study using pramipexole to determine the effectiveness of dopamine agonists in patients with bipolar II depression (Zarate et al. 2004). Subjects on lithium or valproate with therapeutic serum concentrations for at least two weeks were randomly assigned to treatment with pramipexole ($n=10$) or placebo ($n=11$) for 6 weeks. Over the first 5–7 days blinded pramipexole was administered 0.125 mg three times a day and increased every 5–7 days by 0.125 three times a day to achieve the target range of 1.0–3.0 mg/day. The maximum dosage allowable was 4.5 mg/day, and the mean final dosage was 1.7 mg/day. Change from baseline MADRS scores showed a significant treatment effect at week 3 and week 6. Response rates (>50% decrease in MADRS from baseline) were 60% in patients taking pramipexole and 9% in patients taking placebo ($P=0.02$). One subject on pramipexole (who was a responder) and two on placebo (who were nonresponders) developed hypomanic symptoms but completed the trial.

Although these small controlled studies both found adjunctive pramipexole superior to placebo, and provided encouragement for further study, they offer insufficient evidence to establish adjunctive pramipexole as a treatment for bipolar depression, due to the small sample sizes. These double-blind studies are at least as remarkable for the low placebo response rates (20% and 9%) as for the observed benefit of active treatment (67% and 60%). It is not clear to what extent motoric activation or other adverse effects impacted blinding, which becomes very important in small studies like these where, if the ratings for even one subject in each group changed from a responder to a nonresponder or vice versa, the results would no longer be statistically significant.

Omega-3 Fatty Acids

Omega-3 fatty acids, eicosapentaenoic acid (EPA) and docosahexaenoic acid (DHA) are essential nutrients that a preliminary, small, controlled trial suggested might have prophylactic benefit for bipolar disorder (Stoll et al. 1999). That study was undertaken largely on theoretical grounds because in vitro inhibition of phosphokinase-C is a property omega-3 fatty acids share with lithium and valproate. Omega-3 fatty acids also contribute to a range of other physiological processes thought to be relevant to mood regulation (Mirnikjoo et al. 2001). The encouraging preliminary results have not yet been replicated, nor has any form of omega-3 fatty acids demonstrated acute benefit for any aspect of bipolar disorder. The SFBN conducted a double-blind, randomized, placebo-controlled study that failed to show efficacy of omega-3 fatty acids (6 g of EPA or placebo for 4 months) in the treatment of 59 acutely depressed bipolar subjects (Post et al. 2003a). In a small study of depressed unipolar subjects receiving ongoing standard antidepressant treatment, Nemets et al. (2002) found significantly greater reduction in Ham-D scores for those randomized to adjunctive treatment with EPA (1 g, twice daily) compared to placebo. Marangell, however, found DHA (1 g, twice daily) ineffective as monotherapy in a placebo controlled trial for unipolar depression (Marangell et al. 2003). Conceivably, the variance in the results may reflect differences in response between unipolar and bipolar subjects, an effect limited to augmenting standard antidepressants or uncertainty about the correct dosage. Omega-3 fatty acids remain an intriguing, well-tolerated treatment, but still lack proven benefit for bipolar disorder.

Phototherapy

Bright light and dawn simulation have been reported beneficial for some depressed bipolar patients. This is consistent with Winkler and colleagues' finding that among 610 seasonal affective disorder patients, 21.7% suffered from bipolar II disorder, and 1.3% were diagnosed as having bipolar I (Winkler et al. 2002). However, no rigorous, controlled trials have reported results specifically for bipolar depression. Furthermore, bright light alone is seldom sufficient treatment for bipolar depressed patients including those with seasonal pattern (Pjrek et al. 2004). Treatment-emergent hypomania and rarely mania have been reported in response to bright light treatment (Chan et al. 1994).

Magnetic Stimulation

Accumulating evidence associates abnormalities in regional cerebral activity, as indicated by altered blood flow and glucose metabolism in prefrontal and anterior paralimbic basal ganglia-thalamocortical circuits, with the pathophysiology underlying depression and mania. Transcranial magnetic stimulation (TMS) is a novel therapeutic approach available in some research centers. This noninvasive technique can stimulate (at higher frequencies) or inhibit (at lower frequencies) cerebral activity in circuits adjacent to the vicinity of a magnetic stimulator external to the skull. No full scale trails have been reported for bipolar depression, but TMS has been described as beneficial for some cases of bipolar depression (Li et al. 2004; Nahas et al. 2001; Speer et al. 2000).

The optimal parameters for treatment of bipolar depression remain to be established. In addition to location, field strength, and schedule, treatment results appear to vary with the stimulus frequency. Speer reported a double-blind crossover study evaluating the antidepressant effect and changes in regional cerebral blood flow (rCBF) after treatment with 1- and 20-Hz TMS. TMS was administered daily for 2 weeks at 100% of motor threshold over the left prefrontal cortex in 10 depressed subjects (eight unipolar and two bipolar). As hypothesized by the authors, high frequency (20 Hz) TMS over the left prefrontal cortex consistently caused significant increases in rCBF (in prefrontal cortex, the cingulate gyrus, and the left amygdala, as well as bilateral insula, basal ganglia, uncus, hippocampus, parahippocampus, thalamus, and cerebellum). Conversely low frequency (1 Hz) TMS consistently caused significant decreases in rCBF (in small areas of the right prefrontal cortex, left medial temporal cortex, left basal ganglia, and left amygdala). Mood changes following the two TMS frequencies were inversely related ($r=-0.78$, $P<0.005$, $n=10$) such that individuals who improved with one frequency worsened with the other. This apparent demonstration of frequency-dependent, opposite effects of high and low frequency TMS on cerebral activity in circuits adjacent to the vicinity of magnetic stimulation is promising but has not been found consistently (Hoppner et al. 2003). Given the increasing awareness of the importance of variation in stimulation parameters and individual factors, further research is needed as current TMS techniques are likely suboptimal and of limited reliability.

Echo-planar magnetic resonance spectroscopic imaging (EP-MRSI) may represent a therapeutic brain stimulation technique with potential to reliably target stimuli to precisely localized regions more remote to the skull than is possible with TMS. Following anecdotal reports of mood improvement in patients with bipolar disorder immediately after EP-MRSI, researchers at McLean Hospital are investigating EP-MRSI as a therapeutic procedure. Using a scale designed to assess mood states over brief intervals, they report mood improvement in 76.7% of 30 bipolar disorder subjects and 28.6% of 14 healthy comparison subjects who received EP-MRSI versus 30% of 10 bipolar disorder subjects who received sham EP-MRSI (Rohan et al. 2004). The durability and reproducibility of these encouraging results are unknown.

Sleep Deprivation

Mood elevating effects of a night of total sleep deprivation have been reported to be significantly more common in bipolar depression than unipolar depression (Barbini et al. 1998). Unfortunately these effects are generally transient and may precipitate mania (Riemann et al. 2002; Wright 1993). There are no controlled trials, but attempts to sustain the benefit by combining total sleep deprivation with lithium, TMS, bright light, sleep phase advance, or antidepressant medication have had mixed results (Benedetti et al. 2001, 2003).

Risk of Treatment-Emergent Affective Switch

Since bipolar disorder is characterized by an irregular course of recurrent episodes, the occurrence of mania/hypomania, and a substantial proportion of untreated depressions that end with a switch to mania, it is challenging to confidently attribute a switch into mania to any particular event that preceded it.

Antidepressants and Affective Switch and Cycle Acceleration

Concern was raised when Wehr and Goodwin observed apparent shortening of cycle length during periods on antidepressant treatment in a series of 6 bipolar patients (Wehr and Goodwin 1979). Subsequently, Wehr (Wehr et al. 1988) and Koukopoulos (Koukopoulos et al. 2003) also reported a series of rapid-cycling patients in whom onset of rapid cycling was associated with tricyclic antidepressants and resolution of rapid cycling was associated with discontinuation of tricyclic antidepressants. In contrast, recent data from the NIMH National Collaborative Study found rapid cycling resolved within 2 years in 80% of patients but did not find evidence that tapering tricyclic antidepressants was associated with resolution of rapid cycling (Coryell et al. 2003).

Although concerns remain substantial about the potential of standard antidepressants as the cause of mania and cycle acceleration, these phenomena remain to be conclusively established. A large measure of this concern reflects a legacy of observed switches from depression to mania in temporal association with initiation of antidepressant medications and uncontrolled case series which suggest 31%–70% of bipolar patients treated with standard antidepressants alone (that is, in the absence of agents that can prevent mania) will experience TEAS (Goodwin and Jamison 1990). While it is important to understand that data indicating a risk of TEAS associated with antidepressant use was not detected in any rigorous category A studies, it is equally important to understand that no such studies have been specifically designed to assess this issue. Furthermore, it is not prudent to dismiss the risk of TEAS based on meta-analysis of trials intended to obtain regulatory approval that include no formal assessment of abnormal mood elevation (Gijsman et al. 2004; Peet 1994). It is nonetheless fair to say that those trials that have included formal assessment suggesting induction of mania are likely to be limited to a relatively small subgroup of vulnerable patients.

As might be expected, independent of any causal link, the risk of TEAS during antidepressant treatment appears to be reduced by concurrent use of mood stabilizing agents. Most but not all reports suggest the risk of TEAS is greater with tricyclics than other classes of antidepressant medication (Bottlender et al. 2001). Bupropion may be associated with lower rates of switch than desipramine or venlafaxine (Post et al. 2003b; Sachs et al. 1994). As noted above, Vieta also found a fourfold higher switch rate associated with venlafaxine compared to paroxetine (Vieta et al. 2002) and data from STEP-BD suggest prior history of antidepressant associated TEAS is predictive of future risk as is a history of rapid cycling. Bottlender also found an association between risk of TEAS and hypothyroidism (Bottlender et al. 2000b).

The above concerns regarding the potential of standard antidepressants to yield rapid cycling, have fueled research assessing other approaches, such as lithium, divalproex, carbamazepine, lamotrigine, olanzapine, and quetiapine, to treat this subtype of bipolar disorder associated with prominent depressive features (see Chapter 5).

Practical Clinical Strategies for Management of Bipolar Depression

STEP-BD uses clinical treatment pathways to organize a series of critical decisions with recommendations for evidence-based treatment options. Following recognition of a new episode of bipolar depression, the treating psychiatrist and patient confront the 14 basic clinical decision points summarized in Table 3–3. Like all STEP-BD pathways, the bipolar depression pathway begins with assessment and assurance of safety before progressing to initiation of specific acute phase treatment.

Who Should Have Acute Phase Treatment for Depression?

Dysphoria need not meet the 2-week duration criteria for major depression to be dangerous or cause impairment. Transient dysphoric states are common but make a difficult target for pharmacotherapy. Treatments with lag times of 2–12 weeks between initiation and response are far from optimal for patients with acute episode durations substantially shorter than the exposure time required for onset of antidepressant action. Beware of brief and biphasic episodes: the subgroup with well-documented bi-

Table 3–3. Bipolar depression pathway decision points

Decision points	Initial management recommendations
1. Determine need for acute phase antidepressant treatment.	Review symptom acuity and duration of past episodes of depression.
2. Ensure safety.	Choose appropriate treatment venue.
	Acutely depressed patients may require hospitalization.
	Monitor suicidality.
	Initiate medical work up as clinically necessary to rule out life threatening conditions and common causal factors.
	Taper and eliminate if possible use of substances with known depressogenic effects (e.g., sedatives, antihypertensives, steroids, substances of abuse).
3. Menu of Reasonable Choices: Determine the most appropriate regimen for acute treatment.	Sequential care
	Urgent care

Table 3–3. Bipolar depression pathway decision points (*continued*)

Decision points	Initial management recommendations	
4. Initiate/optimize a treatment plan with bimodal (antidepressant and antimanic/prophylactic) properties.	Offer monotherapy treatment with agents having evidence of bimodal activity: lamotrigine, lithium, valproate, olanzapine.	Offer ECT or Offer combination treatment with lamotrigine, lithium, valproate, olanzapine or another agent with proven antimanic or prophylactic activity and an agent with proven efficacy for bipolar depression.
5. Determine indication for dopamine blocking agents (antipsychotic) medication.	Review indication for dopamine blocking agents.	
6. Consider psychosocial intervention with evidence of acute efficacy.	Determine capacity to participate in CBT or another therapy focused on amelioration of acute symptoms.	
7. Offer treatment for comorbid conditions.	Encourage abstinence. Target anxiety symptoms.	

Table 3–3. Bipolar depression pathway decision points *(continued)*

Decision points	Initial management recommendations
8. Determine indication for adjunctive use of agents proven efficacious for unipolar depression.	Review antidepressant Menu of Reasonable Choices.
9. Determine indication for ECT.	Review indications for ECT.
10. Determine indication for nonstandard treatment.	Review Indications for Nonstandard treatments and Innovative treatment options.
11. Determine appropriate follow-up interval.	Schedule follow-up.
12. Determine quantity of medication to be dispensed.	Review potential for overdose, drug interactions, safety in overdose and alternatives for dispensing medication.
13. Consider addition of maintenance phase treatments in the regimen.	See relapse prevention pathway.
14. Has the trial reached a therapeutic endpoint?	Titrate dose to achieve recovery, or declare treatment intolerable or ineffective.
15. Evaluate continuation in pathway.	Exit if meets criteria for mania, hypomania, mixed, or recovered.

phasic episodes in which a depressive phase is followed by a manic or mixed phase without an intervening recovery is particularly worrisome (Zarate et al. 2001). Naturalistic estimates suggest 20%–40% of bipolar patients diagnosed with depression will have a hospitalization or present for outpatient treatment with symptoms of hypomania or mania within 4–8 weeks (Benazzi 2004; Gitlin et al. 2003).

Supportive strategies that ensure safety at the initiation of treatment are an important component of care even for bipolar patients with longer episode durations. Treatments directed at resolution of depression are unlikely to bring substantial relief in less than 4 weeks and may produce increased motivation and motoric mobilization before impacting the morbid thought process and distorted perceptions that make the depressed state dangerous. Throughout this period prior to the expected onset of action, prescribed medications should be presumed inadequate protection for patients at risk unless accompanied by other interventions aimed at controlling distress. Antidepressants now have warnings of their association with treatment-emergent suicidal ideation, a phenomenon of particular concern in children (Healy 2003), as noted in Chapter 6. The risk of self-harm and incapacity associated with bipolar depression may require more frequent outpatient pharmacotherapy and psychotherapy visits, increased family involvement, partial hospitalization, and even inpatient hospitalization until treatment can be safely carried out with the resources available in less restrictive settings. In addition, careful attention to aggressive management of concurrent anxiety disorders and substance abuse can help enhance outcomes of bipolar depression.

Determine the Appropriate Acute Care Strategy

Depending on symptom acuity and therapeutic priorities, specific interventions directed at resolution of the acute symptoms of depression may be initiated using sequential or urgent care strategies. Sequential care gives priority to tolerability and usually involves starting or adding a single intervention initiated at a low dose. Urgent care is necessary when the priority is placed on minimizing the time to onset of symptom relief. Unfortunately, to date there are few controlled data that suggest any specific pharmacological interventions provide an advantage with respect to more rapid onset of action. Although as noted above, olanzapine plus fluoxetine, olanzapine monotherapy, and quetiapine monotherapy separated from placebo by the end of week one in controlled trials, head to head comparisons within the same trial are needed to address this issue. Combining pharmacological, psychological, and family interventions is common in urgent care, although controlled studies are needed to establish the efficacy of such multimodal approaches. With both sequential and urgent care, each treatment trial should be carried out to a meaningful therapeutic endpoint (see below) leading into the relapse prevention pathway, mood elevation pathway, or remaining in the depression pathway for another iteration of acute depression treatment.

Menu of Reasonable Choices: Selection of an Appropriate Initial Treatment Regimen

Most guidelines suggest that initial treatment for bipolar depression should avoid unopposed (in the absence of an agent to prevent mania) antidepressant therapies. A regimen with bimodal therapeutic action can be provided by combining antimanic agents with an antidepressant or by choosing a single treatment with bimodal (antidepressant and antimanic) activity. When agents with only antidepressant activity are administered, bipolar patients should also receive protection against further cycling by treatment with agents with proven acute or prophylactic antimanic activity. While several medications have demonstrated bimodal acute and/or prophylactic activity, none are equally and robustly effective against depression and mania.

Agents with bimodal activity appear to be effective for a substantial proportion of bipolar depressed patients even when used without standard antidepressant medication. In fact, the most methodologically sound trial available that compared a mood stabilizer alone to mood stabilizer and antidepressant found no benefit of the combination over lithium alone (Nemeroff et al. 2001). Naturalistic data from STEP-BD (Sachs 2003b) indicate that response rates for bipolar depression were the same when bimodal agents ("mood stabilizers") were used with or without standard antidepressant medication. Although published reports suggest each of the bimodal agents may be effective at least in open use, lamotrigine, lithium, olanzapine, and quetiapine have the best evidence supporting their utility.

Even when not effective as monotherapy, treatment with bimodal agents may have two other potential benefits. First, these agents may, like lithium, reduce the potential risk of TEAS associated with concomitant antidepressants used by approximately 50% of patients (Prien et al. 1984). Second, in an analysis of data from the double-blind comparison of maintenance treatment with placebo, lithium, and valproate, Gyulai et al. (2003) reported that when dysphoria prompted the open addition of an SSRI, patients maintained on placebo compared to those on divalproex were substantially less successful in averting a full depressive relapse. Thus, combinations of bimodal agents and standard antidepressants may be not only less likely to yield TEAS but also more likely to provide relief of bipolar depression compared to use of standard antidepressants alone. Hence there is some evidence to support expert consensus recommendations to use a bimodal agent in every phase of the illness and avoid monotherapy with standard antidepressants (Keck et al. 2004). When standard antidepressant medications are prescribed, the co-administration of lithium, lamotrigine, valproate, olanzapine, or another agent with antimanic properties is always recommended.

Sequential Care Strategy

In the majority of cases, over the first 3 weeks of treatment it is reasonable to offer patients with mild to moderate bipolar depression a single agent with bimodal activity ("mood stabilizer" medications). If the patient is not substantially improved at that point, sequential addition of standard antidepressants or ECT should be offered unless contraindicated based on individual history.

Urgent Care Strategy

For the most severely ill patients, ECT should be offered as the safest, fastest, and most effective acute treatment available. When this is unacceptable or when tolerability and risk of mania are not of paramount clinical priority, treatment can be initiated with a bimodal agent and a standard antidepressant. Depressed bipolar patients with psychosis, acute suicidal intent, or severe agitation are important candidates for ECT, but may find it more acceptable to begin an alternative urgent care strategy with a combination of bimodal agents, a standard antidepressant, and a dopamine-blocking agent.

Selection of Treatments With Specific Antidepressant Efficacy

Based on data from unipolar depression, the efficacy of approved standard antidepressant medications appears equivalent overall (Frank et al. 1993) and all could be considered for use in treatment of bipolar depression. In constructing the menu of reasonable choices, antidepressant drugs with the most desirable adverse effect profile (very low likelihood of serious adverse effects and very high tolerability of expectable adverse effects) could be considered as potential first-line antidepressant treatment. A menu of reasonable choices for individual cases would be selected from this subset based on the prior treatment history, specific contraindications (allergy, cardiac status, insurance restrictions, cost, safety in overdose), tolerability concerns, and preferences of each patient. ECT and treatments with mechanism of action similar to first-line agents but somewhat less desirable adverse effect profiles are available if preferred based on individual patient factors.

Acute Phase Management After Treatment Initiation

Each acute phase trial that is initiated should be carried out to reach a meaningful therapeutic endpoint: full response, intolerance, or inadequate response. Partial response should be considered a tentative evaluation subject to more definitive reinterpretation in light of further experience at a higher dose or longer treatment duration. The goals of follow-up visits during the acute phase include assuring safety, monitoring response, optimizing therapeutic ef-

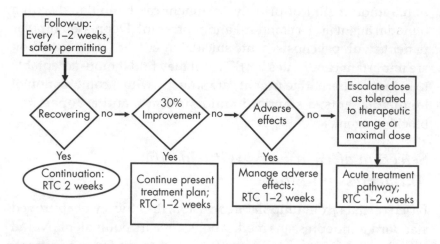

Figure 3–2. Controlled trials for acute bipolar depression, ($n \geq 60$)
Note. RTC=return to clinic

fects, and minimizing adverse effects. Figure 3–2 illustrates decision making over a typical course of acute treatment. When patients experience remission of acute depression it is appropriate to offer continuation treatment. Similarly, in some instances it may be advisable for a time to make no changes in the treatment for patients with substantial improvement (>30%) and receiving maximum tolerated pharmacotherapy, even though their clinical status remains "depressed" or "continued symptomatic." In such instances, more time on the same regimen may yield additional improvement, whereas decreasing or replacing current medications might yield loss of partial responses, and increasing or adding agents could result in unacceptable adverse effects.

Reports from Nierenberg and Fava suggest a progressively lower conditional probability of response given no significant improvement after 2, 4, 6, and 8 weeks of treatment at a given dose of antidepressant medication (Nierenberg et al. 1995). Therefore, patients experiencing no significant improvement and tolerating treatment without significant adverse effects are candidates for upward dose titration until reaching maximal tolerated doses. When adverse effects preclude increasing dosage, titration is delayed or dosage may be decreased to allow management of adverse effects. If these tactics do not suffice to achieve an adequate outcome, alternative treatment may be required. For patients with clear worsening, it is reasonable to cut a trial short and move on to an alternative treatment especially if concern arises that treatment has contributed to the increased dysphoria or worsening of suicidal ideation. Otherwise, patients should be encouraged to sustain treatment at least 6 weeks at an adequate dosage in order to fairly evaluate a treatment trial.

Transition to continuation treatment begins when a clinical status of "recovering" is assigned, but the transition from "recovering" to "recovered" is frequently not smooth. For most patients the early months typically include weeks in which the assigned clinical status will be "continued symptomatic" or "depression." Such full or partial "relapses" are common and when persistent may indicate a need for further titration of acute phase treatment.

Determine Indications for Nonstandard Treatments: Unproven Exploratory Options

The availability of standard agents with differing structures, mechanisms, and adverse effect profiles provides a long list of options, which can be confidently offered before turning to nonstandard treatments. However, there is little to be gained with respect to avoiding adverse effects or avoiding confounding influences of multiple interventions by forbidding patients to use well-tolerated adjuncts such as acupuncture, homeopathy, or dietary supplements with no known contraindications, keeping in mind that even "natural" interventions can result in problems such as TEAS with S-adenyl-methionine (SAM-E), or drug interactions with Saint John's Wort. In contrast, there is much to be lost with respect to the therapeutic alliance, if such adjunctive approaches are prohibited, particularly when suggested or preferred by the patient. In order to assess their impact, exploration of these treatments and response should also be tracked in the chart.

Determine Indication for ECT

ECT may be appropriate at any time, including as an initial treatment when dictated by symptom acuity or patient preference, and all patients should be made aware of its availability. ECT may be encouraged as an early option for acutely suicidal, psychotic, catatonic, or severely depressed patients but is generally held in reserve for patients intolerant of or refractory to mood stabilizers and standard antidepressant medications. As noted in Chapter 7, ECT may be an important treatment option in pregnancy, especially in cases of suicidal or homicidal ideation (infanticide) or psychotic decompensation. Ethical considerations suggest all patients using refractory to standard bimodal agents in combination with a standard antidepressant be reminded of ECT as a treatment option.

Determine Indication for Antipsychotic Medication

Patients with delusions, hallucinations, and severe agitation often benefit from adjunctive antipsychotic medications. Atypical antipsychotic medication may improve some symptoms of depression but there are no direct comparison data as yet suggesting that these agents have antidepressant properties comparable to standard antidepressant medications. Atypical antipsychotics are preferred over older (neuroleptic/conventional) antipsychotics, as the latter appear more implicated in causing neurological adverse effects and, particularly at a high dosage, can increase dysphoria in some patients.

Determine Follow-up Intervals

Local standards and clinician judgment determine acceptable intervals for follow-up. In most circumstances when new medical treatment is initiated, a follow-up interval of 1–2 weeks is appropriate for managing most outpatients. Patients with mild to moderate depression and good support systems may be more safely managed at longer intervals than severely ill patients who lack reliable supports, but all depressed patients are at risk for self-destructive behavior. In the absence of reliable predictors of dangerousness, it is important to evaluate both inclination and opportunity for self-harm. Patients with active suicidal ideation or other signs of high inclination (such as comorbid anxiety, substance use, or history of suicide attempts) warrant aggressive treatment aimed at reducing symptoms of depression and of comorbid conditions, and may require hospitalization, since none of the currently available antidepressant treatments for outpatients deliver reliable results in less than 3 weeks. If measures are taken to adequately monitor the patient and reduce opportunities for self-harm (e.g., eliminate access to firearms and other lethal agents), many acutely depressed patients can be managed without hospitalization, particularly if family/social supports are mobilized. Accordingly, it is best to initiate treatment with a follow-up interval that avoids dispensing large amounts of potentially lethal medications (especially lithium and tricyclic antidepressants).

Determine Quantity of Medication to be Dispensed

Depression is a risk factor for suicide even in patients evidencing no current self-destructive urges. Limiting the quantity of medication prescribed at any one time to amounts that would not be lethal if ingested in their entirety does not by itself assure safety, but can lessen one potential source of lethality. Dispensing amounts of medication sufficient to ensure supply to the next appointment may require extra safety measures, such as having a family member involved in the control of the patient's medications.

Endpoints

Acute phase treatment of bipolar depression continues unless the patient experiences affective switch (hypomanic, manic, mixed episode) or meets recovery criteria. Patients who are unable to tolerate an effective dosage or are unresponsive to a full trial of maximal dose are offered acute treatment with another standard antidepressant, ECT, or innovative treatment depending on their symptom acuity and history of prior response. Before concluding that a treatment is ineffective, some experts recommend augmentation strategies such as lithium, thyroid, stimulants, or neurotransmitter precursors in efforts to potentiate standard treatments. The benefits of many such interventions are not well established, but augmentation strategies may be beneficial even if their contribution is limited to sustaining therapeutic optimism and the therapeutic alliance long enough to complete a 6-week therapeutic trial with the highest tolerated dosage of a standard agent.

Management of treatment-emergent affective switch begins with informing patients and family members of the risk of switch and warning signs. There are no category A data to guide management of TEAS, but reduction or elimination of antidepressant medication may be sufficient management in some mild cases. Treatment is otherwise the same as primary hypomania or mania.

Considerations for Special Subpopulations

The subpopulation of treatment-naïve bipolar I and bipolar II patients includes a substantial proportion of good prognosis patients likely to respond well to bimodal agents. Patients with a history of treatment and who are suffering a recurrence during an interval in which they received no prophylactic treatment are also frequently responsive to mood stabilizer treatment.

Patients with breakthrough episodes occurring during ongoing maintenance treatment appear to be less treatment responsive, particularly if the breakthrough occurred while receiving therapeutic levels of lamotrigine, lithium, valproate, olanzapine, or carbamazepine. Such patients may, however, respond to an increased dosage of their prophylactic treatment aimed at improving the antidepressant benefit of bimodal agents, particularly if their medication was maintained at suboptimal levels (e.g., lithium <0.8 mMol/L, lamotrigine <200 mg/day, valproate <80 µg/mL, olanzapine 10 mg/day, quetiapine <300 mg/day, or carbamazepine <8.0 µg/mL).

Breakthrough episodes occurring during the course of prophylaxis with bimodal agents and standard antidepressants may represent an even more refractory subgroup but might also include some cases in which the course of illness was driven by the antidepressant itself (El-Mallakh and Karippot 2002). For these patients, recommendations for acute treatment follow the same guideline (increase dose or add a new antidepressant) but following appropriate continuation treatment, unsuccessful acute treatments, and those ineffective for prophylaxis would be tapered in the maintenance phase. Careful record keeping is necessary to ascertain the effects of treatments that are sustained in the maintenance phase.

Patients with a history of TEAS or rapid cycling are at highest

risk to experience treatment-emergent switch or cycle acceleration when treated with standard antidepressants, and may benefit from the alternative approaches described in Chapter 5.

Conclusions

Treatment of acute episodes of bipolar depression has long been
a matter of debate in which options for intervention were often
selected on the basis of opinion informed by little high quality evidence. The past 5 years has brought not only an increase in the
number of studies addressing treatment for bipolar depression
but also an encouraging increase in the quality of available data.
Our expanded fund of knowledge brings psychiatric practice to
an era in which it is possible to apply the principles of evidence-
based medicine to the treatment of bipolar depression.

The morbidity and mortality associated with bipolar depression present a compelling humanitarian rationale for the administration of aggressive treatment. Concerns about efficacy and the
potential for TEAS continue to cast an inadequately characterized but worrisome shadow over the use of standard antidepressant medications that have gained wide acceptance for the
treatment of unipolar depression. There are, however, few adequate data demonstrating the benefit of exposing patients to
many of the standard antidepressant medications traditionally
regarded as first-line interventions for bipolar depression. Quantitative data from well designed controlled trials helps put these
concerns in perspective. The available evidence does not support
routinely withholding standard antidepressants from the treatment of bipolar II patients or bipolar I patients receiving concurrent therapies with antimanic properties. However, naturalistic
effectiveness data from the Stanley Research Network and STEP-
BD suggest only about 15%–25% of depressed bipolar subjects
treated with a standard antidepressant medication will meet recovery criteria. Furthermore, even among the fortunate minority
meeting the recovery criteria, 20%–25% relapsed within
4 months, regardless of whether or not antidepressant medication was continued (Altshuler et al. 2003; Sachs 2003b). Nevertheless, a small minority of patients who tolerate and respond to

adjunctive antidepressants may do better if these agents are continued rather than discontinued. The evidence from controlled trials of antidepressant efficacy supporting lamotrigine, olanzapine, and quetiapine now supports the consideration of these agents as first-line treatments of bipolar depression. These and other novel interventions offer encouragement that better alternatives will become available in the future.

References

Altshuler L, Suppes T, Black D, et al: Impact of antidepressant discontinuation after acute bipolar depression remission on rates of depressive relapse at 1-year follow-up. Am J Psychiatry 160(7):1252–1262, 2003

American Psychiatric Association: Practice guideline for the treatment of patients with bipolar disorder (revision). Am J Psychiatry 159 (suppl 4):1–50, 2002

Amsterdam J: Efficacy and safety of venlafaxine in the treatment of bipolar II major depressive episode. J Clin Psychopharmacol 18(5):414–417, 1998

Amsterdam JD, Garcia-Espana F, Fawcett J, et al: Efficacy and safety of fluoxetine in treating bipolar II major depressive episode. J Clin Psychopharmacol 18(6):435–440, 1998

Amsterdam JD, Schults J, Brunswick DJ, et al: Short-term fluoxetine monotherapy for bipolar type II or bipolar NOS major depression— low manic switch rate. Bipolar Disord 6(1):75–81, 2004

Ballenger JC, Post RM: Carbamazepine in manic-depressive illness: a new treatment. Am J Psychiatry 137(7):782–790, 1980

Barbini B, Colombo C, Benedetti F, et al: The unipolar-bipolar dichotomy and the response to sleep deprivation. Psychiatry Res 79(1):43–50, 1998

Benazzi F: Intra-episode hypomanic symptoms during major depression and their correlates. Psychiatry Clin Neurosci 58(3):289–94, 2004

Benedetti F, Campori E, Barbini B, et al: Dopaminergic augmentation of sleep deprivation effects in bipolar depression. Psychiatry Res 104(3):239–246, 2001

Benedetti F, Colombo C, Serretti A, et al: Antidepressant effects of light therapy combined with sleep deprivation are influenced by a functional polymorphism within the promoter of the serotonin transporter gene. Biol Psychiatry 54(7):687–692, 2003

Black DW, Winokur G, Nasrallah A: ECT in unipolar and bipolar disorders: a naturalistic evaluation of 460 patients. Convuls Ther 2(4):231–237, 1986

Bottlender R, Jager M, Strauss A, et al: Suicidality in bipolar compared to unipolar depressed inpatients. Eur Arch Psychiatry Clin Neurosci 250(5):257–261, 2000a

Bottlender R, Rudolf D, Strauss A, et al: Are low basal serum levels of the thyroid stimulating hormone (b-TSH) a risk factor for switches into states of expansive syndromes (known in Germany as "maniform syndromes") in bipolar I depression? Pharmacopsychiatry 33(2):75–77, 2000b

Bottlender R, Rudolf D, Strauss A, et al: Mood-stabilisers reduce the risk of developing antidepressant-induced maniform states in acute treatment of bipolar I depressed patients. J Affect Disord 63(1–3):79–83, 2001

Bryant-Comstock L, Stender M, Devercelli G: Health care utilization and costs among privately insured patients with bipolar I disorder. Bipolar Disord 4(6):398–405, 2002

Cade J: Lithium salts in the treatment of psychotic excitement. Med J Aust 2:249–352, 1949

Calabrese JR, Bowden CL, Sachs GS, et al: A double-blind placebo-controlled study of lamotrigine monotherapy in outpatients with bipolar I depression. Lamictal 602 Study Group. J Clin Psychiatry 60(2):79–88, 1999

Calabrese J, Macfadden W, McCoy R, et al. Double-blind placebo-controlled study of quetiapine in bipolar depression. Paper presented at the 157th annual meeting of the American Psychiatric Association. New York, May 2004a

Calabrese JR, Kasper S, Johnson G, et al: International consensus group on bipolar I depression treatment guidelines. J Clin Psychiatry 65(4):571–579, 2004b

Cassano P, Lattanzi L, Soldani F, et al: Pramipexole in treatment-resistant depression: an extended follow-up. Depress Anxiety 20(3):131–138, 2004

Chan PK, Lam RW, Perry KF: Mania precipitated by light therapy for patients with SAD. J Clin Psychiatry 55(10):454, 1994

Cohn JB, Collins G, Ashbrook E, et al: A comparison of fluoxetine imipramine and placebo in patients with bipolar depressive disorder. Int Clin Psychopharmacol 4(4):313–322, 1989

Coryell W, Solomon D, Turvey C, et al: The long-term course of rapid-cycling bipolar disorder. Arch Gen Psychiatry 60(9):914–920, 2003

Daly JJ, Prudic J, Devanand DP, et al: ECT in bipolar and unipolar depression: differences in speed of response. Bipolar Disord 3(2):95–104, 2001

Davis LL, Bartolucci A, Petty F: Divalproex in the treatment of bipolar depression: a placebo controlled study. J Affect Dis, in press

Dunner DL, Stallone F, Fieve RR: Lithium carbonate and affective disorders. V: A double-blind study of prophylaxis of depression in bipolar illness. Arch Gen Psychiatry 33(1):117–120, 1976

El-Mallakh RS: An open study of methylphenidate in bipolar depression. Bipolar Disord 2(1):56–59, 2000

El-Mallakh RS, Karippot A: Use of antidepressants to treat depression in bipolar disorder. Psychiatr Serv 53(5):580–584, 2002

Fieve RR, Platman SR, Plutchik RR: The use of lithium in affective disorders. I. Acute endogenous depression. Am J Psychiatry 125(4):487–491, 1968

Frank E, Karp JF, Rush AJ: Efficacy of treatments for major depression. Psychopharmacol Bull 29(4):457–475, 1993

Frye MA, Ketter TA, Kimbrell TA, et al: A placebo-controlled study of lamotrigine and gabapentin monotherapy in refractory mood disorders. J Clin Psychopharmacol 20(6):607–614, 2000

Ghaemi SN, Rosenquist KJ, Ko JY, et al: Antidepressant treatment in bipolar versus unipolar depression. Am J Psychiatry 161(1):163–165, 2004

Gijsman HJ, Geddes JR, Rendell JM, et al: Antidepressants for bipolar depression: a systematic review of randomized, controlled trials. Am J Psychiatry 161(9):1537–1547, 2004

Gitlin M, Boerlin H, Fairbanks L, et al: The effect of previous mood states on switch rates: a naturalistic study. Bipolar Disord 5(2):150–152, 2003

Goldberg JF, Burdick KE, Endick CJ: Preliminary randomized, double-blind, placebo-controlled trial of pramipexole added to mood stabilizers for treatment-resistant bipolar depression. Am J Psychiatry 161(3):564–566, 2004

Goodwin F, Jamison K: Manic Depressive Illness. New York, Oxford University Press, 1990

Goodwin GM: Evidence-based guidelines for treating bipolar disorder: recommendations from the British Association for Psychopharmacology. J Psychopharmacol 17(2):149–173, 2003

Gyulai L, Bowden CL, McElroy SL, et al: Maintenance efficacy of divalproex in the prevention of bipolar depression. Neuropsychopharmacology 28(7):1374–1382, 2003

Healy D: Lines of evidence on the risks of suicide with selective serotonin reuptake inhibitors. Psychother Psychosom 72(2):71–79, 2003

Himmelhoch JM, Thase ME, Mallinger AG, et al: Tranylcypromine versus imipramine in anergic bipolar depression. Am J Psychiatry 148(7):910–916, 1991

Hlastala SA, Frank E, Mallinger AG, et al: Bipolar depression: an underestimated treatment challenge. Depress Anxiety 5(2):73–83, 1997

Hoppner J, Schulz M, Irmisch G, et al: Antidepressant efficacy of two different rTMS procedures. High frequency over left versus low frequency over right prefrontal cortex compared with sham stimulation. Eur Arch Psychiatry Clin Neurosci 253(2):103–109, 2003

Joffe RT, Uhde TW, Post RM, et al: Motor activity in depressed patients treated with carbamazepine. Biol Psychiatry 22(8):941–946, 1987

Joffe H, Hall JE, Cohen LS, et al: Polycystic ovarian syndrome associated with valproate in women with bipolar disorder. Paper presented at the annual meeting of the American Psychiatric Association, New York, May 2004

Judd LL, Akiskal HS, Schettler PJ, et al: The long-term natural history of the weekly symptomatic status of bipolar I disorder. Arch Gen Psychiatry 59(6):530–537, 2002

Judd LL, Akiskal HS, Schettler PJ, et al: A prospective investigation of the natural history of the long-term weekly symptomatic status of bipolar II disorder. Arch Gen Psychiatry 60(3):261–269, 2003

Keck PE Jr, Perlis RH, Otto MW, et al: The expert consensus guideline series: treatment of bipolar disorder 2004. Postgrad Med (Spec):1–120, 2004

Koukopoulos A, Sani G, Koukopoulos AE, et al: Duration and stability of the rapid-cycling course: a long-term personal follow-up of 109 patients. J Affect Disord 73(1–2):75–85, 2003

Kupfer DJ, Chengappa KN, Gelenberg AJ, et al: Citalopram as adjunctive therapy in bipolar depression. J Clin Psychiatry 62(12):985–990, 2001

Kupfer DJ, Frank E, Grochocinski VJ, et al: Demographic and clinical characteristics of individuals in a bipolar disorder case registry. J Clin Psychiatry 63(2):120–125, 2002

Lambert PA, Carraz G, Borselli S, et al: Neuropsychotropic action of a new anti-epileptic: depemide. Ann Med Psychol Paris 124:707–710, 1966

Lambert PA, Venaud G: Use of valpromide in psychiatric therapeutics. Encephale 13(6):367–373, 1987

Li X, Nahas Z, Anderson B, et al: Can left prefrontal rTMS be used as a maintenance treatment for bipolar depression? Depress Anxiety 20(2):98–100, 2004

Marangell LB, Martinez JM, Zboyan HA, et al: A double-blind, placebo-controlled study of the omega-3 fatty acid docosahexaenoic acid in the treatment of major depression. Am J Psychiatry 160(5): 996–998, 2003

McIntyre RS, Mancini DA, McCann S, et al: Topiramate versus bupropion SR when added to mood stabilizer therapy for the depressive phase of bipolar disorder: a preliminary single-blind study. Bipolar Disord 4(3): 207–213, 2002

McIntyre RS, Mancini DA, Lin P, et al: Treating bipolar disorder. Evidence-based guidelines for family medicine. Can Fam Physician 50:388–94, 2004

Mendlewicz J, Youdim MB: Antidepressant potentiation of 5-hydroxytryptophan by L-deprenil in affective illness. J Affect Disord 2(2):137–146, 1980

Mirnikjoo B, Brown SE, Kim HF, et al: Protein kinase inhibition by omega-3 fatty acids. J Biol Chem 276(14):10888–10896, 2001

Murphy DL, Goodwin FK, Brodie HK, et al: L-dopa, dopamine, and hypomania. Am J Psychiatry 130(1):79–82, 1973

Nahas Z, Teneback CC, Kozel A, et al: Brain effects of TMS delivered over prefrontal cortex in depressed adults: role of stimulation frequency and coil-cortex distance. J Neuropsychiatry Clin Neurosci 13(4):459–470, 2001

Nemeroff CB, Evans DL, Gyulai L, et al: Double-blind, placebo-controlled comparison of imipramine and paroxetine in the treatment of bipolar depression. Am J Psychiatry 158(6):906–912, 2001

Nemets B, Stahl Z, Belmaker RH: Addition of omega-3 fatty acid to maintenance medication treatment for recurrent unipolar depressive disorder. Am J Psychiatry 159(3):477–479, 2002

Nierenberg AA, McClean NE, Alpert JE, et al: Early nonresponse to fluoxetine as a predictor of poor 8-week outcome. Am J Psychiatry 152(10):1500–1503, 1995

Ostroff RB, Nelson JC: Risperidone augmentation of selective serotonin reuptake inhibitors in major depression. J Clin Psychiatry 60(4):256–259, 1999

Peet M: Induction of mania with selective serotonin re-uptake inhibitors and tricyclic antidepressants. Br J Psychiatry 164(4):549–550, 1994

Perugi G, Toni C, Ruffolo G, et al: Adjunctive dopamine agonists in treatment-resistant bipolar II depression: an open case series. Pharmacopsychiatry 34(4):137–141, 2001

Pjrek E, Winkler D, Stastny J, et al: Bright light therapy in seasonal affective disorder—does it suffice? Eur Neuropsychopharmacol 14(4):347–351, 2004

Post RM, Uhde TW, Roy-Byrne PP, et al: Antidepressant effects of carbamazepine. Am J Psychiatry 143(1):29–34, 1986

Post RM, Altshuler LL, Frye MA, et al: Rate of switch in bipolar patients prospectively treated with second-generation antidepressants as augmentation to mood stabilizers. Bipolar Disord 3:259–265, 2001

Post RM, Leverich GS, Altshuler LL, et al: An overview of recent findings of the Stanley Foundation Bipolar Network (Part I). Bipolar Disord 5(5):310–319, 2003a

Post RM, Leverich GS, Nolen WA, et al: A re-evaluation of the role of antidepressants in the treatment of bipolar depression: data from the Stanley Foundation Bipolar Network. Bipolar Disord 5(6):396–406, 2003b

Prien RF, Kupfer DJ, Mansky PA, et al: Drug therapy in the prevention of recurrences in unipolar and bipolar affective disorders: report of the NIMH Collaborative Study Group comparing lithium carbonate, imipramine, and a lithium carbonate-imipramine combination. Arch Gen Psychiatry 41(11):1096–1104, 1984s

Prudic J, Sackeim HA, Devanand DP: Medication resistance and clinical response to electroconvulsive therapy. Psychiatry Res 31(3):287–296, 1990

Prudic J, Olfson M, Marcus SC, et al: Effectiveness of electroconvulsive therapy in community settings. Biol Psychiatry 55(3):301–312, 2004

Riemann D, Voderholzer U, Berger M: Sleep and sleep-wake manipulations in bipolar depression. Neuropsychobiology 45 (suppl 1):7–12, 2002

Rohan M, Parow A, Stoll AL, et al: Low-field magnetic stimulation in bipolar depression using an MRI-based stimulator. Am J Psychiatry 161(1):93–98, 2004

Royal Australian and New Zealand College of Psychiatrists Clinical PRactice Guidelines Team for Deliberate Self-Harm: Australian and New Zealand clinical practice guidelines for the treatment of bipolar disorder. Aust N Z J Psychiatry 38(5):280–305, 2004

Sachs G: Mood stabilizers versus standard antidepressants for treatment of bipolar depression. Paper presented at the annual meeting of the American College of Neuropsychopharmacology. San Juan, Puerto Rico, December 2003a

Sachs GS: STEP-BD update: what have we learned, in International Bipolar Disorder. Pittsburgh, PA, Western Psychiatric Institute and Clinic, UPMC Health System, 2003b

Sachs G: Strategies for improving treatment of bipolar disorder: integration of measurement and management. Acta Psychiatr Scand 422:7–17, 2004

Sachs GS, Lafer B, Stoll AL, et al: A double-blind trial of bupropion versus desipramine for bipolar depression. J Clin Psychiatry 55(9):391–393, 1994

Sachs G, Collins MA, Altshuler LL, et al. Divalproex sodium versus placebo for treatment of bipolar depression. Paper presented at the annual meeting American College of Neuropharmacology. San Juan, Puerto Rico, Decemeber 2001

Sachs GS, Thase ME, Otto MW, et al: Rationale, design, and methods of the systematic treatment enhancement program for bipolar disorder (STEP-BD). Biol Psychiatry 53(11):1028–1142, 2003

Shopsin B, Gershon S: Dopamine receptor stimulation in the treatment of depression: piribedil (ET-495). Neuropsychobiology 4(1):1–14, 1978

Silverstone T: Moclobemide versus imipramine in bipolar depression: a multicentre double-blind clinical trial. Acta Psychiatr Scand 104(2):104–109, 2001

Silverstone PH, Silverstone T: A review of acute treatments for bipolar depression. Int Clin Psychopharmacol 19(3):113–24, 2004

Speer AM, Kimbrell TA, Wassermann EM, et al: Opposite effects of high and low frequency rTMS on regional brain activity in depressed patients. Biol Psychiatry 48(12):1133–1141, 2000

Stoll AL, Severus WE, Freeman MP, et al: Omega-3 fatty acids in bipolar disorder: a preliminary double-blind, placebo-controlled trial. Arch Gen Psychiatry 56(5):407–412, 1999

Tohen M, Vieta E, Calabrese J, et al: Efficacy of olanzapine and olanzapine-fluoxetine combination in the treatment of bipolar I depression. Arch Gen Psychiatry 60(11):1079–1088, 2003

Truman C, Baldassano CF, Goldberg JF, et al: Self-reported treatment-emergent affective switch associated with antidepressant use in the STEP 500. Paper presented at the APA Ninth Annual Research Colloquium for Junior Investigators, New York, May 2004

Wehr T, Goodwin FK: Tricyclics modulate frequency of mood cycles. Chronobiologia 6(4):377–385, 1979

Wehr TA, Sack DA, Rosenthal NE, et al: Rapid cycling affective disorder: contributing factors and treatment responses in 51 patients. Am J Psychiatry 145(2):179–184, 1988

Winkler D, Praschak-Rieder N, Willeit M, et al: Seasonal affective depression in two German speaking university centers: Bonn, Vienna. Clinical and demographic characteristics. Nervenarzt 73(7):637–643, 2002

Winsberg ME, DeGolia SG, Strong CM, et al: Divalproex therapy in medication-naïve and mood-stabilizer-naive bipolar II depression. J Affect Disord 67(1–3):207–212, 2001

Worthington JJ 3rd, Kinrys G, Wygant LE, et al: Aripiprazole as an augmentor of selective serotonin reuptake inhibitors in depression and anxiety disorder patients. Int Clin Psychopharmacol 20(1):9–11, 2005

Wright JB: Mania following sleep deprivation. Br J Psychiatry 163:679–680, 1993

Vieta E, Martinez-Aran A, Goikolea JM, et al: A randomized trial comparing paroxetine and venlafaxine in the treatment of bipolar depressed patients taking mood stabilizers. J Clin Psychiatry 63(6):508–512, 2002

Young LT, Joffe RT, Robb JC, et al: Double-blind comparison of addition of a second mood stabilizer versus an antidepressant to an initial mood stabilizer for treatment of patients with bipolar depression. Am J Psychiatry 157(1):124–126, 2000

Zarate CA Jr, Tohen M, Fletcher K: Cycling into depression from a first episode of mania: a case-comparison study. Am J Psychiatry 158(9):1524–1526, 2001

Zarate CA Jr, Payne JL, Singh J, et al: Pramipexole for bipolar II depression: a placebo-controlled proof of concept study. Biol Psychiatry 56(1):54–60, 2004

Zornberg GL, Pope HG Jr: Treatment of depression in bipolar disorder: new directions for research. J Clin Psychopharmacol 13(6):397–408, 1993

Chapter 4

Long-Term Management of Bipolar Disorder

Charles L. Bowden, M.D.
Vivek Singh, M.D.

Bipolar disorder is a complex, chronic, recurrent illness associated with serious individual and societal costs including increased health care costs, decreased productivity and functioning, poor quality of life, and an increased risk of suicide (Calabrese and Shelton 2002; Goodwin 2002). However, despite our understanding of the chronic and lifelong nature of this illness, treatments often have been short-term and episode focused.

The past decade has seen major paradigm shifts in the treatment of bipolar disorder—acute to maintenance treatment, focus on the illness rather than episodes, and a focus on "functional recovery" rather than mere "syndromal recovery." These three shifts form the core principles in the long-term management of bipolar illness. They have occurred because of a realization of 1) the chronic nature of the illness, interspersed by "crises" involving acute episodes of mania, depression, and mixed states that are similar to the hypertensive crises seen in hypertension; and because of 2) a lag in improvement of socio-occupational functioning among patients despite symptomatic recovery.

Maintenance treatment of bipolar disorder is best accomplished with an approach that combines pharmacological and psychosocial interventions. Pharmacotherapy involves using medications that, alone or in combination, prevent the occurrence of new episodes; facilitate socio-occupational functioning by minimizing the number and intensity of interepisode symptoms; and are devoid of intolerable side effects, thus facilitating long-term compliance with the medication regimen. Remission of symptoms and more importantly "functional recovery"—the primary goals of treatment—are attainable despite the complex and chronic nature of bipolar disorder.

Principles of Long-Term Management

Focus on Long-Term Compliance

Bipolar disorder requires lifelong management because it is a lifelong illness. Ninety percent of patients will experience a recurrence of manic episodes. It has been shown that probability of response to lithium, but not to valproate, is inversely proportional to the number of lifetime episodes (Gelenberg et al. 1989; Swann et al. 1999), which emphasizes the importance of preventing episodes. A maintenance study involving lithium and divalproex sodium demonstrated a substantial reduction in total treatment costs in patients who took medications for 3 months or longer as compared with patients who discontinued their medications prior to 3 months (Revicki et al. 2003). A higher rate of relapse with subsequent need for inpatient treatment accounted for the majority of the difference in cost between the two groups. A large study involving bipolar I patients demonstrated that the average length of continuous lithium treatment was only 65 days (Johnson and McFarland 1996), despite the prophylactic benefit of lithium. These data and the recurrent nature of this illness indicate a need to facilitate compliance with long-term pharmacotherapy.

Compliance is greatly influenced by the adverse effect profile of medications used; thus, choosing medications or combinations of medications with benign adverse effect profiles will enhance tolerability and compliance. Lithium, despite its prophylactic benefits, can make long-term compliance challenging because it can yield many adverse effects and has a low safety index. Lithium and divalproex sodium at serum levels of 0.8 mEq/L and 45 µg/mL or higher, respectively, are effective in the treatment of acute bipolar I mania (Bowden and Gonzales 2001). The frequency and intensity of adverse effects of these two medications are a direct function of their serum levels (Bowden 2001; Gelenberg et al. 1989; Vestergaard et al. 1998). Some patients, particularly those with the "softer spectrum of bipolar disorder," may do well with lower dosages of lithium or valproate and possibly other drugs as well (Jacobsen 1993).

However, a recent analysis of a 1-year randomized treatment study with either divalproex or lithium found that bipolar I patients whose serum valproate levels were maintained between 75 and 99 μg/mL had significantly better outcomes than did patients with either lower or higher serum drug levels (Keck et al. 2002) (see Table 4–1 and Figure 4–1). This study suggested that efforts to further improve response by increasing divalproex to achieve levels greater than 100 μg/mL for maintenance therapy is unlikely to be efficacious. In contrast, responses to established sub-therapeutic, low therapeutic, mid-therapeutic, and high therapeutic serum levels of lithium differed neither from each another nor from placebo. Thus, although there are reasons to keep serum lithium levels below those associated with adverse effects, there may be patients who respond to lithium in ways subtly related, or even unrelated, to serum levels maintained. Compliance can be enhanced by minimizing the emergence of adverse effects and with skillful management strategies such as using sustained-release preparations to minimize peak levels (and hence adverse effects); using once-a-day dosing; closely monitoring for adverse effects; lowering dosage; optimizing dosage or serum concentration of one medication, if tolerated, before adding another drug to avoid unnecessary polypharmacy; and using lower dosages of drugs with tolerability limitations in combination with another drug (Muller-Oerlinghausen et al. 2000; Sachs et al. 2002; Tohen et al. 2003b). If a medication is inadequately tolerated, or simply ineffective, it should be discontinued and alternative regimens should be implemented.

Denial of the severity of illness is another reason for poor compliance (Scott and Pope 2002). Patients' unwillingness to accept that they have bipolar disorder or that their illness requires treatment greatly affects their attitudes toward their illness and can lead to behaviors that negatively affect compliance (Scott and

Table 4–1. Median survival time: discontinuation for protocol-defined mania or depression

Treatment group (*N*)	Median survival time, months (95% confidence limit)
Placebo (88)	3.5 (2, 5)
Lithium	
Nontherapeutic (5)	1 (1, 3)
Low therapeutic (16)	4 (2, 10)
Medium therapeutic (37)	4 (2, 9)
High therapeutic (16)	3 (1, 5)
Divalproex	
Nontherapeutic (11)	5 (1, NC)
Low therapeutic (45)	5 (4, 10)
Medium therapeutic (85)	8 (5, 12)
High therapeutic (28)	2 (1, 3)

Note. NC= not calculable.

Pope 2002). This is most often a problem early in the course of illness and can be addressed in part with psychoeducational programs. In addition, some patients mistakenly perceive symptom-free periods as evidence of "cure" and hence a signal to discontinue further treatment. Establishment of a therapeutic alliance through regular visits and an empathic collaborative approach will help overcome illness denial and resistance to treatment. Education of the patient and family of the chronic nature of the illness and involvement of the family in clinical care also may improve compliance (Colom et al. 2003a, 2003b).

Recognizing "Signal Events"

We define *signal events* as events or behaviors that indicate a patient either 1) has returned to a baseline level of functioning or 2) is at risk of a relapse or recurrence. Recognition of these events or behaviors helps focus on the current clinical state and tailor the treatment to meet the needs of the patient. For example, return of mild irritability, agitation, or insomnia may be the harbinger of a manic episode and an indication of the need for medication ad-

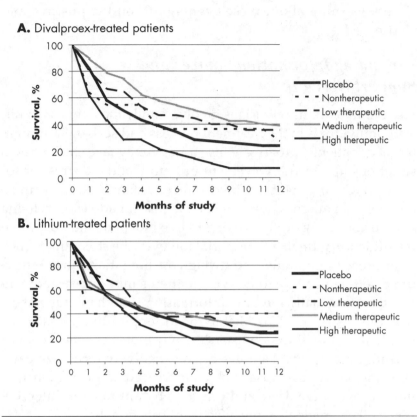

A. Divalproex-treated patients

B. Lithium-treated patients

Figure 4–1. Survival analysis: different patterns of discontinuation for any reason with varying plasma drug concentrations.

Kaplan-Meier survival curves for divalproex-treated patients (A) and lithium-treated patients (B) who were discontinued from the double-blind treatment period of the study for any reason. Only divalproex at the medium therapeutic concentration range demonstrated a statistically significant difference ($P<0.05$) from placebo.

justment. Similarly, the return of interest in hobbies, such as gardening, music, or sports, previously enjoyed by the patient may be a "signal" that the depressive episode is in remission. These behaviors or events may not be recognized or reported by the patient and may be missed even by an astute clinician. A therapeutic relationship, based on empathy, collaboration, and trust, will facilitate patients' reporting these symptoms to their psychiatrists. Collateral information from patients' families will also facilitate learning about these events both on the positive and alerting sides.

Expanding Information Sources and Support Network

We recommend that clinicians involve family members or significant individuals in the treatment process and seek their input in terms of patients' progress. This strategy may face challenges in situations in which involvement of family adds to stress or for patients who may perceive involvement of family as an infringement of their autonomy, as may be the case for adolescents living at home or young adults seeking to live independently of parental influence or financial support. However, the strengths of such an approach commonly far outweigh the limitations. In the structured setting of a brief office visit, patients may appear more intact than is actually the case. Information from family members that reflects the patients' behavior in longitudinal, less structured, more stressful circumstances, may more accurately convey current illness state. Families often sensitively recognize early warning signs of relapse such as increased self-confidence or more provocative dress and can thereby aid in early interventions to keep patients more effectively functional.

Involvement of families provides clinicians opportunities to assess and address family expectations. If these are unrealistic, families can be worked with to develop more realistic expectations based on improved understanding of the goals of treatment and prognosis of the illness. Families can also aid in providing structured settings for patients and financial and emotional support that can positively affect prognosis.

Treatment Strategies for Common Events During Maintenance Care

Worsening depression is much more common than worsening mania during prophylaxis, particularly so among patients whose most recent syndromal episode was depressive (Calabrese et al. 2003a). (Chapter 3 in this volume discusses acute bipolar depression in detail.) The most common intervention, based on numerous reviews, may be one of the least efficacious: use of an antidepressant without a mood stabilizer (Altshuler et al. 1995). Among a group of poorly responding patients, antidepressant therapy without mood stabilizers was associated with unsuccessful outcomes in 80%. The only blinded, randomized data come from a study of divalproex, lithium, and placebo. The time to development of depressive symptoms requiring intervention was significantly longer for patients randomized to divalproex than either to placebo or lithium. Once a selective serotonin reuptake inhibitor (SSRI) was added, both the divalproex plus SSRI combination and the lithium plus SSRI combination resulted in longer time in study than an SSRI as monotherapy. An analysis of time to dropout for depression showed that less than 10% of the patients given divalproex plus SSRI failed, compared with 45% of the patients given an SSRI alone, with intermediate benefits from the lithium plus SSRI regimen.

Among the small subset of patients who obtain benefit without mood destabilization for 6 months from addition of antidepressants to mood stabilizers, those who continue on the antidepressants for 1 year may have better outcomes than those tapered off antidepressants (Altshuler et al. 2003). In aggregate, studies conclusively indicate that antidepressants alone are inadequate treatments for emergent acute depression in bipolar disorder but that mood stabilizer plus antidepressant combinations can be efficacious and well tolerated for some patients. These findings suggest that recommendations to halt an adjunctive antidepressant as soon as depression is alleviated are probably unwarranted in patients who do not experience mood destabilization on these agents. combined with mood stabilizers.

The recent lamotrigine studies in maintenance treatment indicate that lamotrigine is effective in reducing the likelihood of depressive relapse over time. Interestingly, the greatest advantage of lamotrigine over placebo was among recently manic patients, for whom fewer than 20% even required an intervention for depression over an 18-month period (Bowden et al. 2003). These data suggest a useful strategy may be adding lamotrigine as part of a prophylactic regimen in all bipolar I patients, regardless of episode type. Lamotrigine was well tolerated by patients when added to lithium or divalproex during the acute phase (Keck et al. 2002; Metz et al. 2002). Lamotrigine was least effective in those patients with histories of severe depression, suggesting that even for a drug established as effective, more aggressive regimens may be needed for patients with the most severe depressions (Bowden, in preparation). Long-term data for lamotrigine in combination with other drugs are generally limited to case reports and uncontrolled studies, and controlled studies are needed.

Spotlight on the Illness

Treatment of bipolar disorder should focus on the management of a chronic illness rather than merely controlling syndromal episodes. Bipolar patients, even when in remission, continue to experience subthreshold or minor symptoms between episodes, including cognitive dysfunction (Martinez-Aran et al. 2004). Persistence of subthreshold symptoms, but not relapse into new episodes, may be a stronger predictor of poor functional outcome (Gitlin et al. 1995). Moreover, functional recovery commonly lags behind syndromal recovery by several months (Horgan 1981; Tohen et al. 2000). Clinicians must carefully monitor and manage subthreshold symptoms to improve both socio-occupational functioning and quality of life.

A focus on the illness will help identify symptoms during the "infancy stage" that may precede full-blown episodes. Early intervention, by preventing full-blown episodes and possible hospitalization, will help control financial costs, because most health care costs in the management of this illness come from inpatient treatment and emergency department visits. We recommend that patients be closely monitored, through regular visits, even during periods of remission.

Identification and Modification of Risk Factors for Relapse

Clinicians must identify factors or conditions that may increase the risks of relapse or emergence of new episodes or worsen the course of the illness, particularly ones that are modifiable. Mania,

Table 4–2. Common medical conditions that can precipitate mania

Stroke	Sleep deprivation
Traumatic brain injury	Wilson's disease
Hyperthyroidism	Multiple sclerosis
Vitamin B_{12} deficiency	Epilepsy
Cushing's disease	HIV infection
Herpes simplex	AIDS
Uremia	Systemic lupus erythematosus

mixed mania, and hypomania share common risk factors for relapse. Therefore, in this discussion we use the term *mania* to imply all three states.

Comorbid General Medical Illness

Comorbid medical conditions, some of which are listed in Table 4–2, can precipitate a manic episode and, if untreated, may lead to long-term worsening of the illness (Goldberg 1998). Thus treatment of these medical conditions should go hand in hand with management of bipolar illness. Communication among the psychiatrists, other physicians, and allied mental health professionals on the patient's treatment team is strongly recommended.

Medications/Illicit Drugs

Table 4–3 lists common medications/illicit drugs that could precipitate mania in patients with bipolar illness (Goldberg 1998). Most bipolar patients have a current or prior history of alcohol or substance abuse problems. Educating patients and families of the inherent mood-destabilizing effects of these substances is critical. A comprehensive treatment plan should be developed to concurrently address both bipolar illness and substance abuse/dependence problems. Clinicians should inquire of their patients all medications that they are currently taking, at each visit, including over-the-counter and herbal remedies, to check for potential drug–drug interactions and to identify any medications that may yield mood destabilization.

Table 4–3. Mood destabilizing medications/illicit drugs

Alcohol	Antidepressants,
Bronchodilators	particularly tricyclics
Caffeine	Hallucinogens
Cocaine	Interferon
Stimulants	Dopamine agonists
Steroids	Pseudoephedrine

Pregnancy and Postpartum Period

As noted in Chapter 7 by Rasgon and Zappert, pregnancy and the postpartum period are crucial times with respect to choice of treatment (especially during pregnancy, to attenuate or avoid the risks of birth defects with pharmacotherapy) and risk of relapse (especially during the postpartum period, which entails a high risk of relapse). In many instances clinicians, patients, and their families have to choose between challenging options, such as determining whether to accept the risks of treating (birth defects) or not treating (emergent episodes) during pregnancy. At such times an empathic collaborative approach to making risk-management decisions is essential.

Sleep

Sustained lack of sleep over several days has the potential to precipitate manic, hypomanic, or mixed episodes (Goodwin and Jamison 1990). Although a single night of total or repeated nights of partial sleep deprivation may transiently counter depressive symptoms, such interventions (particularly when repeated for days on end) entail the risk of mood destabilization. Professions that require long work hours or shift work, such as law enforcement, health care, or other emergency work, can put bipolar patients at risk for manic relapse or mood destabilization. Similarly, sleep difficulties associated with the last trimester of pregnancy and the postpartum period increase the risk of relapse. Helping patients maintaining sleep regularity with behavioral (teaching sleep hygiene) and if needed pharmacological approaches can help reduce the risk of manic relapses.

Stress

Stress can increase the risk of mood instability in patients with bipolar illness. The exact mechanism for this phenomenon is not known, but it is hypothesized that stress activates the autonomic system and causes dysregulation of the hypothalamic-pituitary-adrenal (HPA) axis, causing bipolar patients to have manic relapses. This may also explain the higher prevalence of HPA dysfunction in mixed manic states (Evans and Nemeroff 1983; Krishnan et al. 1983; Swann et al. 1990).

Light

Increased exposure to light has a propensity to precipitate mania in patients with bipolar disorder. Summer may predispose patients to the risk of a manic relapse, whereas autumn can precipitate depressive episodes (Silverstone et al. 1995). Exposure to artificial light and travel between time zones that extends the period of light exposure may lead to manic relapse. Whether the risk of relapse is simply due to a function of sleep disruption or due to a dysregulation of circadian pacemaking or neurotransmitters such as melatonin or serotonin (which may be in involved in the etiology of bipolar disorder) remains to be established. Educating patients about these modifiable risk factors can be instrumental in maintaining mood stability.

Fostering a Therapeutic Alliance

Bipolar disorder is a complex, chronic, lifelong illness that, although inherited, is strongly influenced by the external milieu. An illness of such nature requires a strong therapeutic relationship between the treating clinician and the patient. Systematic data regarding the impact of psychosocial factors or any specific psychotherapeutic approach on the course of illness in bipolar disorder are only beginning to emerge. Compliance with treatment, a primary objective of treatment, is positively affectedby counseling (Miklowitz and Goldstein 1990). A recent randomized study determined that a combination of family-focused therapy and pharmacotherapy for bipolar patients led not only to a reduction in mood symptoms but also to better medication adherence compared with pharmacotherapy plus less intensive crisis management intervention (Miklowitz et al. 2003).

Establishment of a therapeutic alliance encourages patients to learn about their illness in an environment that is perceived as safe and structured. This helps clinicians overcome the barriers of denial and resistance to treatment. An empathic collaborative approach, the cornerstone of a therapeutic relationship, helps patients identify the physician as caring and competent and someone that can be trusted in times of crises. It also encourages them to be compliant with treatment, including taking their medications, reporting symptoms and side effects, keeping appointments, and translating their understanding of the illness into everyday life.

Adjunctive Psychological Therapies in Maintenance Treatment

Since 1999, several randomized, controlled studies that have used psychoeducational models have demonstrated the significant benefits of adjunctive psychoeducational therapies beyond those yielded by usual medication management together with outpatient supportive care. Each of the studies has added the psychoeducational approaches to standard medication regimens. The first study of 69 patients at high risk for relapse of bipolar disorder had 6 to 12 sessions of cognitive and behavioral techniques to identify and manage early warning signs of relapse (Perry et al. 1999). Over the course of 18 months of follow-up, the group receiving adjunctive psychoeducation had significantly fewer manic relapses (27% versus 57%), fewer days in the hospital, and longer time between episodes. There were no differences in rates of depressive relapses. In the largest study to date, Colom and associates randomly assigned 120 patients to either 20 sessions of adjunctive group psychoeducation or to an unstructured support group (Colom et al. 2003a). The group receiving adjunctive psychoeducation experienced significantly fewer relapses into mania, mixed mania, or depression.

Controlled studies of adjunctive, technique-driven, psycho-social interventions have also been conducted. Cognitive therapy plus mood stabilizer(s) was superior to usual support plus mood stabilizer(s) in reduction of manic and depressive episodes, but not mixed episodes (Lam et al. 2003). The group receiving adjunctive cognitive therapy also had greater improvement in social adjustment and evidenced better coping strategies for managing prodromal symptoms of mania. In a smaller study of adjunctive family therapy, 31 patients who received 21 sessions of family therapy had fewer relapses and longer delays before relapses compared to 70 patients who received two sessions of family psychoeducation and follow-up crisis management (Miklowitz et al. 2000). Patients who were living in environments of high expressed emotion appeared most likely to benefit. Adjunctive interpersonal and social rhythm therapy appeared to improve social rhythms (e.g., time of going to bed) compared to intensive clinical management. However, no differences in time to remission were observed. Among the subset of patients who entered the study in a depressive episode, time to recovery with adjunctive interpersonal psychotherapy was briefer (Hlastala et al. 1997).

These consistently positive results are still undergoing more detailed analyses. It appears that efforts to help patients recognize early signs of illness are more effective for the manic side of the illness than for the depressive side. This may be attributable to evidence that manic relapses tend to develop over longer time frames than do depressive relapses, and that many manic symptoms are qualitatively different from ordinary experiences, whereas depressive symptoms tend to be quantitatively greater, but not qualitatively different (Jackson et al. 2003). There is some developing evidence that the benefits of these techniques are largely limited to patients with greater social supports and less severe forms of bipolar disorder. Although the studies have tended to be technique-driven, there are several features shared by the specific brief therapies including attention to medication compliance, identifying early signs of episodes, improving coping skills, involvement of significant others, and provision of information about the features, course, and treatment of bipolar disorders.

Long-Term Pharmacotherapy in Bipolar Disorder

General Principles

Evidence-based treatment guidelines for the long-term management of bipolar disorder are only beginning to emerge. This is a function of the small number of long-term placebo-controlled studies performed in bipolar disorder, most likely related to ethical, logistical, and financial issues. Because bipolar disorder is a multidimensional illness, placebo-controlled studies have one inherent drawback: lack of generalizability to the full spectrum of the illness (Baldessarini et al. 2000; Bowden et al. 2000). In this section we also discuss data from open label trials and active comparator trials to further aid in developing management recommendations.

The first 6 months account for the largest differences among treatment reponses in bipolar patients being treated with mood stabilizers (Bowden et al. 2000; Coryell et al. 1997). Treatments beyond this time frame are essentially similar in terms of rates of relapse or improvement in symptoms. Poor compliance due to adverse effects, commonly associated with long-term treatment, may be responsible for the lack of difference between treatments beyond 6 months, although studies are needed to assess this phenomenon.

Because compliance with treatment greatly determines long-term outcome, it is essential to use medications that have the largest probability of being not only effective but also well tolerated. The probability of discontinuation of medications or noncompliance is commonly a direct function of the severity and frequency of adverse effects associated with the medications. Strategies to maximize compliance include using the least number of medications at the lowest dosages while optimizing effectiveness; educating patients about the role of each medication and its side effects; aggressively managing emergent side effects; and using lower dosages of medications in combinations to minimize side effects. Medications with inherent mood-destabilizing properties such as antidepressants, which are used adjunctively in acute depressive episodes, should be used at the least effective dosage and should be tapered and discontinued following improvement, particularly if there is personal current or prior evidence of mood destabilization with these agents. However, a minority of bipolar disorder patients who respond to and tolerate antidepressants combined with mood stabilizers may benefit from ongoing combination therapy (Altshuler et al. 2003). Tricyclic antidepressants, possibly due to their effects on a greater number of neurotransmitters involved in the pathogenesis of depressive episodes, appear more likely than the newer antidepressants, such as the SSRIs or buproprion, to cause mood instability (Altshuler et al. 2003).

Lithium

Lithium was the first drug approved by the U.S. Food and Drug Administration (FDA) for the maintenance treatment of bipolar disorder. Double-blind, placebo-controlled trials conducted in the 1970s, using lithium either as monotherapy or in combination with other agents, showed a significant difference in the rates of relapse between lithium and placebo groups—34% versus 87%, respectively (Goodwin 2002). The unusually high placebo relapse rate in the studies may have been due to abrupt discontinuation of stable dosages of lithium prior to randomization (Moncrieff 1995).

In a randomized, open comparison of lithium and carbamazepine, lithium proved to have superior efficacy and tolerability than carbamazepine (Greil et al. 1997). However, these differences emerged when criteria for efficacy was broadened to include development of new episodes, need for additional medications, or hospitalization. Also, subsequent analysis revealed subgroup differences. Thus, maintenance treatment with lithium was more effective than carbamazepine in patients with "classical" bipolar disorder (bipolar I disorder with no mood-incongruent delusions or comorbidity) but tended to be more effective with carbamazepine than lithium in patients with "non-classical" bipolar disorder (bipolar II disorder, bipolar disorder not otherwise specified, bipolar disorder with mood-incongruent delusions or comorbidity; Greil et al. 1998).

In another study, lithium maintenance treatment appeared

more effective than carbamazepine in patients with no more than 6 months' prior exposure to either agent (Hartong et al. 2003). However, this advantage was offset by more early discontinuations in the lithium group, so that similar proportions (about one-third) of patients completed 2 years with no episode. Patients given lithium compared with those given carbamazepine tended to have somewhat greater risk of episodes in the first 3 months and markedly less risk of episodes afterward, with a recurrence risk of only 10% per year with lithium after the first 3 months. Patients given carbamazepine had a more consistent rate of relapse/recurrence of about 40% per year.

Marginal efficacy and low rates of continuation with lithium treatment were noted in open studies done in the 1990s (Coryell et al. 1997; Gitlin et al. 1995; Harrow et al. 1990; Maj et al. 1998; Vestergaard et al. 1998). The lower rates of efficacy of lithium were related to its poor tolerability and consequently poor compliance. Some patients, however, did well on long-term treatment with lithium and the rates of suicide and suicidal behaviors were seven- to eightfold (Goodwin 2002) lower in patients treated with lithium compared with those who were untreated.

The efficacy of lithium is more pronounced in certain subtypes of bipolar patients, including those with euphoric mania, family history of bipolar disorder, an episode sequence of mania-depression-euthymia, and periods of complete remission of symptoms between episodes (Goodwin 2002). On the other hand, patients with rapid cycling, higher numbers of depressive or manic episodes, mixed states or dysphoric mania, comorbid substance abuse, secondary mania, and psychotic symptoms tend to respond more poorly to lithium (Goodwin 2002).

Lithium, in three blinded, randomized studies (Bowden et al. 2000; Denicoff et al. 1997; Dunner et al. 1976), proved to be an effective agent for management of manic symptoms but allowed worsening of depressive symptoms. This was clearly demonstrated in two recent randomized, placebo-controlled trials involving lithium and lamotrigine. The studies showed lithium and lamotrigine were significantly superior to placebo in time to prolonging intervention for any mood episode, the primary efficacy measure. Lithium, however, was significantly more effective than placebo in prolonging time to intervention for manic, mixed, or hypomanic episodes but not for depressive episodes (Bowden et al. 2003; Calabrese et al. 2003b). These results are at variance with the widely held belief that lithium is effective as an antidepressant for maintenance treatment and indicate that changing to an alternative mood stabilizer or augmenting with another treatment is helpful if depressive symptoms do not respond to treatment with lithium or if the patient has a relapse or recurrence of a depressive episode.

Clinicians need to educate patients regarding the risk of rapid relapse if lithium is abruptly discontinued (Bowden and Gonzales 2001). Patients on long-term treatment with lithium are likely to discontinue lithium due to 1) intolerable adverse effects, 2) impulsivity and risk-taking behavior, 3) inability to perceive illness as lifelong, and 4) perceiving symptom remission as cure.

There are limited data regarding optimal dosage and serum levels of lithium required for maintenance therapy. Lower rates of relapse (but more adverse effects) have been noted when serum lithium level was maintained between 0.8 mEq/L and 1.0 mEq/L as compared with levels of 0.4–0.6 mEq/L (Gelenberg et al. 1989). Most patients in the lower-level range (0.4–0.6 mEq/L) who relapsed were those in whom lithium dosages were reduced at the time of entry into the study from higher levels on which the psychiatrist had previously maintained them. Patients whose serum levels of lithium were in the 0.4–0.6 mEq/L range prior to randomization had low relapse rates regardless of assignment to either of those two groups (Perlis et al. 2004). Another study noted that serum lithium levels maintained higher than 0.5 mEq/L were associated with lower rates of hospitalization (Maj et al. 1998). Given these data, we recommend serum levels of lithium be maintained at 0.6–0.8 mEq/L during maintenance treatment in many instances. However, lowering of the dosage of lithium is recommended if adverse effects become problematic. In contrast, occasional patients require and can tolerate somewhat higher lithium blood concentrations (0.8–1.0 mEq/L) in maintenance therapy.

Valproate

Valproate has a role in the maintenance treatment of bipolar disorder as evidenced by three randomized studies. The first study

(Lambert and Venaud 1992) compared lithium with an amide form of valproate (valpromide) in 150 patients and noted that the rate of new episodes was 20% lower in patients given valpromide than in those given lithium. The study also showed that patients treated with lithium were more likely to discontinue their medications, either due to lack of efficacy or adverse effects. However, an open label design and inclusion of patients with unipolar recurrent depression limited the conclusiveness of these results.

Bowden et al. (2000) conducted a randomized, double-blind, placebo-controlled, parallel group 12-month maintenance study comparing lithium to divalproex in patients with bipolar I disorder. The three groups did not differ on the primary measure of outcome—time to relapse for any mood episode. However, it was noted that divalproex was superior to placebo on the following secondary outcome measures: proportion of patients who maintained response after 1 year (41% to 13%), mean number of days in treatment (209 versus 143), and proportion of patients discontinuing for relapse (71% versus 50%). This study was limited by the inclusion of a large number of patients with a milder form of the illness and by its use of higher serum levels of both the study drugs (valproate 71–125 mg/L, lithium 0.8–1.2 mEq/L). A recent 47-week study compared valproate with olanzapine for maintenance treatment in bipolar patients with an index episode of acute mania. Patients whose acute mania had responded to either of the agents in a 3-week inpatient trial were included in the study. The two groups did not significantly differ in the rates of manic relapse or in the median time to a manic relapse (Tohen et al. 2003b). Olanzapine was somewhat more poorly tolerated due to sedation, weight gain, and increased cholesterol but was somewhat more effective on some secondary outcome measures.

It is clear that the maintenance efficacy of valproate monotherapy is insufficient, although clinically important, for the majority of patients with bipolar disorder. There have been two randomized, controlled trials comparing the efficacy of valproate in combination therapy with monotherapy with another mood stabilizer. In a small pilot study, when valproate was used in combination with lithium for continuation and maintenance treatment (Solomon et al. 1997), it was noted that this combination was more effective (less relapse or recurrence) but less well tolerated (more adverse effects). An 18-month study comparing the maintenance efficacy of a combination of olanzapine plus lithium or valproate with lithium, or valproate monotherapy (Tohen et al. 2004) demonstrated the superior efficacy of combination treatment. Patients given combination treatment had a longer period to recurrence of mania compared with monotherapy (362 versus 63 days) and lower mania recurrence rate (15% versus 35%).

Carbamazepine

There is a lack of conclusive evidence from randomized, double-blind, placebo-controlled studies for the role of carbamazepine in maintenance treatment of bipolar disorder (Post et al. 1997). For example, an open, randomized maintenance study comparing the efficacy of carbamazepine and lithium found lithium to be superior to carbamazepine except in patients with the atypical forms of mania, who tended to respond better to carbamazepine. In another study, lithium and carbamazepine in combination were more effective than either of these two agents alone on measure of functional improvement (Denicoff et al. 1997). Adverse events involving the dermatological and neuromuscular systems and cognitive side effects are a function of dosage titration and improve with sustained treatment and stabilization of carbamazepine dosage. As noted earlier, randomized trials suggest that lithium may be generally more effective than carbamazepine for maintenance therapy (Greil et al. 1997; Hartong et al. 2003), although some patients with "non-classical" bipolar disorder may tend to respond better to carbamazepine (Greil et al. 1998).

Lamotrigine

Lamotrigine has expanded treatment options in bipolar disorder and was only the second agent approved by the FDA for maintenance treatment in bipolar disorder. Two recently published studies documented the efficacy of lamotrigine for maintenance treatment of bipolar I disorder. The first (Bowden et al. 2003) was a double-blind, placebo-controlled, multicenter trial involving

175 patients that was designed to evaluate the efficacy and tolerability of lamotrigine and lithium compared with placebo for preventing relapse or recurrence of any mood episode in bipolar I patients who were recently manic or hypomanic. Following an open-label phase of 8–16 weeks during which patients were started on lamotrigine and taken off other psychotropics, patients were randomized to lamotrigine, lithium, or placebo for as long as 18 months. Both lamotrigine and lithium were more effective than placebo in prolonging time to intervention for any mood episode. Although lamotrigine was superior to placebo in prolonging time to a depressive episode, lithium was more effective in prolonging time to a manic, hypomanic, or mixed episode.

The second study, which had a similar design, randomized 463 recently depressed patients to lamotrigine, lithium, or placebo (Calabrese et al. 2003a). Both lamotrigine and lithium were superior in efficacy to placebo for prolonging time to intervention for any mood episode. Lamotrigine was significantly more effective than placebo in prolonging time to intervention for depression but not for a manic episode. Lithium, on the other hand, was significantly superior to placebo in prolonging time to intervention for a manic episode but not for depression.

When a combined analysis of data from the two studies was performed, lamotrigine and lithium were superior to placebo in extending time to intervention for any mood episode (Goodwin et al. 2004). Lamotrigine was significantly more effective in prolonging time to intervention for a depressive episode, whereas both lamotrigine and lithium were statistically superior to placebo in prolonging time to intervention for a manic episode.

Open lamotrigine has also been effective as monotherapy and add-on therapy in both bipolar I and bipolar II disorder for up to 48 weeks (Calabrese et al. 1999a, 1999b). As noted in Chapter 5, lamotrigine was also superior on most measures of efficacy, as compared with placebo, in a 26-week randomized, double-blind, placebo-controlled study in patients with rapid-cycling bipolar disorder (Calabrese et al. 2000).

Lamotrigine has not been associated with episode switches or cycle acceleration in placebo-controlled trials and has an adverse effect profile similar to placebo (Calabrese et al. 2003a). The most

Table 4–4.   Dosing guidelines for initiation of lamotrigine

	Lamotrigine alone	Lamotrigine + valproate	Lamotrigine + carbamazepine
Weeks 1 and 2	25 mg/day	25 mg every other day	25 mg twice a day
Weeks 3 and 4	50 mg/day	25 mg/day	50 mg twice a day
Week 5	100 mg/day	50 mg/day	100 mg twice a day
Week 6	200 mg/day	100 mg/day	150 mg twice a day
Week 7			200 mg twice a day

common adverse effect noted was headache. Lamotrigine has minimal impact on weight, cognition, or sexual functioning and does
not require serum monitoring. Calabrese et al. (2003a) published
an analysis of the rates of rash in 12 multicenter clinical trials involving lamotrigine. Of the 3,153 patients exposed to lamotrigine,
11.6% developed a benign rash, whereas less than 0.1% developed
a serious rash. However, in controlled settings the incidence of
rash was lower (lamotrigine 8.3% and placebo 6.4%) and no case of
serious rash occurred. We recommend a gradual titration of lamotrigine to minimize the risk of rash—25 mg/day for the first
2 weeks, 50 mg/day for weeks 3 and 4, and then increasing by 50–
100 mg/week to 200 mg/day or as clinically indicated. If lamotrigine is part of a combination regimen involving carbamazepine, an
inducer of hepatic metabolism, the above dosages should be doubled. On the other hand, for use with valproate, an enzyme inhibitor, we recommend that the starting dosage and titration dosages
of lamotrigine be halved (See Table 4–4).

Antipsychotics

Antipsychotics are frequently used in the treatment of bipolar
disorder. Most patients started on antipsychotics as adjunctive
treatment for manic episodes continue these agents beyond
6 months, even in the absence of conclusive data on the long-

term efficacy of most antipsychotics in maintenance treatment (Kusumakar 2002).

Typical antipsychotics are effective antimanic agents but appear less effective than lithium, valproate, and carbamazepine in the maintenance treatment of bipolar disorder (Kusumakar 2002). Long-term treatment with typical antipsychotics can precipitate depressive episodes (Ahlfors et al. 1981). These data and the greater risk of tardive dyskinesia in affective disorder limit the role of typical antipsychotics for maintenance treatment.

Atypical or novel antipsychotics have a more benign adverse effect profile, and emerging evidence suggests that they may be important options in the treatment of bipolar disorder. As noted in Chapter 2 by Ketter and associates, these agents as a class appear to be effective in acute mania, with olanzapine, risperidone, quetiapine, ziprasidone, and aripiprozole having received FDA indications for acute mania. In addition, as described in Chapter 3, the combination of olanzapine and fluoxetine has been approved by the FDA for the treatment of bipolar depression. Moreover, olanzapine has received FDA approval for maintenance treatment in bipolar disorder, and emerging data suggest that aripiprazole may have efficacy in maintenance therapy. Taken together, this evidence suggests that atypical antipsychotics may ultimately prove to have roles in managing not only acute mania but also acute depression and maintenance therapy in patients with bipolar disorders.

Olanzapine has received an FDA indication not only as an antimanic agent but also for maintenance therapy. Multicenter, randomized, double-blind, placebo-controlled trials indicate that olanzapine as maintenance monotherapy for bipolar disorders after acute manic episodes was superior to placebo (Tohen et al. 2003a) and comparable (and on some measures superior) with lithium (Tohen et al. 2003c). In these studies, olanzapine tended to robustly prevent mania and more modestly prevent depression. Mean olanzapine dosages in these monotherapy maintenance trials after acute manic episodes were approximately 12–16 mg/day, and sedation and weight gain were the main adverse effects. There are only limited data regarding the efficacy of olanzapine as continuation and maintenance therapy after acute depressive episodes in bipolar disorders. In a 52-week continuation study, approximately three-quarters of patients who remitted in an 8-week acute depression study who were placed on open olanzapine monotherapy required addition of open fluoxetine, and even with this intervention allowed, about 45% relapsed (primarily into depression) (Ketter et al. 2004). As noted earlier, in an active-comparator trial, olanzapine monotherapy compared with divalproex monotherapy was somewhat more poorly tolerated due to sedation and weight gain but somewhat more effective on some secondary outcome measures (Tohen et al. 2003b).

Sedation and weight gain are the main adverse effects seen with olanzapine. These difficulties are particularly challenging during maintenance therapy. Increasing concerns have been raised regarding the risks of obesity and diabetes with olanzapine and other newer antipsychotics. Indeed, the FDA has stipulated changes in the product information for not only olanzapine but also other newer antipsychotics to reflect these risks, suggesting a class effect for such problems. In contrast, the report of a recent consensus development conference on antipsychotics and obesity, diabetes, and hyperlipidemia emphasized differences between agents, with clozapine and olanzapine being the most, risperidone and quetiapine being less, and ziprasidone and aripiprazole being the least implicated (American Diabetes Association et al. 2004).

Like other newer antipsychotics, aripiprazole appears effective in acute mania. Multicenter, randomized, double-blind, placebo-controlled trials indicate that aripiprazole monotherapy is effective for acute manic and mixed episodes, and it received such an indication in 2004. In addition, in a recent 26-week double-blind, placebo-controlled trial, aripiprazole was effective as continuation/maintenance treatment in patients with recent manic or mixed episodes, with anxiety and nervousness being the main adverse effects (Keck et al. 2004b). Indeed, aripiprazole received a maintenance indication in early 2005.

To date, there are no controlled trials of risperidone for maintenance therapy in bipolar disorders. However, in a 6-month multicenter study in 541 patients (430 completers) with bipolar disorders or schizoaffective disorder bipolar type, open adjunctive risperidone (mean dosage approximately 4 mg/day) was generally well tolerated, with sedation, weight gain, and extrapyramidal symptoms being the main adverse events (Vieta et al. 2001). In this study, extrapyramidal symptom ratings decreased from baseline to endpoint, and there were no new cases of tardive dyskinesia. Also, in an uncontrolled trial, open risperidone showed benefits when added to patients' medication regimen in treatment that lasted an average of 6 months (Kusumakar 2002).

To date, there are no double-blind, placebo-controlled trials of quetiapine maintenance therapy in bipolar disorders, although small longer-term open treatment trials suggest that open quetiapine is well tolerated in bipolar disorders (Altamura et al. 2003; Suppes et al. 2004).

To date, there are no controlled trials of ziprasidone for acute bipolar depression or maintenance treatment in bipolar disorders. However, open continuation/maintenance studies suggest that ziprasidone is well tolerated and lacks substantial sedation, weight gain, or cardiac problems (Keck et al. 2004a; Weisler et al. 2004).

Clozapine may have utility in bipolar disorder patients. An open, randomized study suggested that adjunctive clozapine was effective in the maintenance treatment of patients with treatment-resistant bipolar and schizoaffective disorder (Suppes et al. 1999). However, the risks of sedation, weight gain, and aplastic anemia, and the inconvenience of frequent blood monitoring for blood dyscrasias, suggest clozapine ought to be held in reserve for patients with treatment-resistant bipolar disorders.

Taken together, these data suggest a possible emerging role for the use of atypical antipsychotics in the maintenance treatment of patients with bipolar disorders. These drugs do not appear to entail as much risk of tardive dyskinesia or exacerbation of depression as seen with typical antipsychotics. However, at least some atypical antipsychotics have been associated with problematic sedation, weight gain, and metabolic disturbances. In addition, further studies are needed to establish whether or not atypical antipsychotics as a class have efficacy in the maintenance treatment of patients with bipolar disorders. Patients whose bipolar disorder is resistant to mood stabilizers or combinations thereof are reasonable candidates for ongoing treatment with atypical antipsychotics, as noted in the 2002 revision of the American Psychiatric Association's practice guideline for bipolar disorders (American Psychiatric Association 2002). Additional controlled studies are needed to clarify the role(s) of atypical antipsychotics in maintenance treatment in patients with bipolar disorders. In the interim, careful assessment of the risks and benefits is indicated before long-term treatment with these agents is pursued.

Antidepressants

Antidepressants are the most commonly prescribed agents in bipolar disorder, despite the very limited studies evaluating their long-term efficacy (Kusumakar 2002). Chapter 3 discusses the use of antidepressants in bipolar depression in detail. Tricyclic antidepressants have proven ineffective in maintenance treatment and may cause switching and cycle acceleration. Controlled studies assessing the newer antidepressants for maintenance treatment have not been undertaken. A recently published study (Altshuler et al. 2003) revealed that in patients who had responded to and tolerated antidepressant augmentation, discontinuing antidepressants within 6 months of remission yielded higher risk of depressive relapse than continuing these agents for longer than 6 months. However, the study was neither blinded nor randomized and only about 15% (84/549) of patients exposed to antidepressants were included in the study. It may be that a small subgroup of bipolar patients do well on maintenance treatment with antidepressants combined with mood stabilizers.

Combination Treatment

Recent 12- to 18-month randomized, controlled studies of lithium, divalproex, lamotrigine, or olanzapine monotherapy have all suggested that no more than about 30% of patients who start maintenance treatment with one medication maintain relatively good control of their illness, avoid new episodes, or do not discontinue treatment early, principally in relationship to side effects. Naturalistic studies also suggest that most patients with bipolar disorder require more than one medication to manage their illness (Levine et al. 2000). Thus, although a small subset of patients do well with maintenance monotherapy for bipolar disorder, most patients clearly do not. In addition to difficulties with tolerability of full-dosage monotherapies, the multidimensional nature of bipolar disorder almost certainly is a factor in the limited efficacy of monotherapy. Studies by Swann et al. (2001, 2002) and others indicate that bipolar disorder is composed of at least four, and possibly six, dimensions or relatively discrete symptom areas. These domains include hyperactivity, impulsivity, depression-anxiety, psychosis, irritability, and grandiosity. Mood stabilizers employed in bipolar disorder have differing efficacy in providing control, or relapse prevention, for these various domains.

As suggested in Chapter 2, the most substantive evidence for efficacy of combination therapies comes from a series of acute mania studies, all published since 2000, that show a mood stabilizer, usually lithium or valproate, plus an antipsychotic to be more effective than the mood stabilizer alone, and vice versa. Thus, divalproex or lithium combined with newer antipsychotics, such as olanzapine (Tohen et al. 2002), risperidone (Sachs et al. 2002; Yatham et al. 2003), and quetiapine (DelBello et al. 2002; Yatham et al. 2004), proved superior to divalproex or lithium combined with placebo in acute mania. In another controlled study, combining valproate with antipsychotics (primarily haloperidol and/or perazine) compared with placebo plus antipsychotics enhanced acute antimanic responses and resulted in lower antipsychotic dosages (Muller-Oerlinghausen et al. 2000). Importantly, the dosage of the added medication was commonly lower than that for monotherapy. Although fewer efficacy studies of combination therapy in maintenance therapy have been published, there are plausible reasons to expect the same favorable profile of action as has been seen consistently in acute episode studies.

As noted earlier, in a small pilot study, divalproex added to lithium for which patients were unresponsive gave improved efficacy (but poorer tolerability) compared with simply continuing lithium monotherapy (Solomon et al. 1997). Also, in patients with treatment-resistant bipolar or schizoaffective disorder, clozapine added to usual therapy—generally involving lithium treatment—was more effective than randomized, but open continuation of the treatment as usual (Suppes et al. 1999).

In the first blinded test of the efficacy of antidepressant monotherapy for breakthrough depression, Gyulai et al. (2003) reported that monotherapy with either paroxetine or sertraline was ineffective in controlling depression and helping patients to complete 1 year of maintenance treatment. In contrast, addition of either SSRI to divalproex was efficacious and significantly superior to monotherapy with SSRIs, both alleviating depression and allowing completion of the maintenance year. Lithium plus SSRI appeared intermediate between SSRI alone and divalproex plus SSRI but was generally closer in effectiveness to the divalproex combination.

As noted previously, a recent 18-month study showed that olanzapine plus either lithium or valproate was superior to either mood stabilizer alone in delaying time to any relapse or delaying time to manic relapse. However, the combination regimen was not significantly superior in delaying time to depressive relapse (Tohen et al. 2004). Importantly, the design of this study involved a sample substantially enriched for olanzapine plus mood stabilizer response. Patients had to have developed manic episodes while taking either lithium or valproate and thus were nonresponders to monotherapy with either agent. Additionally, to be eligible for randomization, the subset of randomized patients who showed the superior efficacy of combination treatment were required to have achieved both syndromal and symptomatic recovery on the olanzapine plus mood stabilizer combination treatment. Less than one-third of patients achieved this high degree of acute manic response. Therefore, combination therapy of an antipsychotic plus a mood stabilizer may be beneficial for a small subset of bipolar patients.

Another reason for combining treatments in maintenance is symptom driven complex clinical states. For example, patients may have achieved generally good mood stability with a single mood stabilizer but may still have sleep disturbance characteristic of bipolar disorder, with increasing energy in the evenings, late time of getting to sleep, reduced total sleep time, and some reversal of day/night schedule. Benzodiazepines or their equivalents or antipsychotic drugs with sedative properties may be preferable as additions for these patients rather than increases in the dosage of the mood stabilizer. Similar rationales apply to addition of medications for control of anxiety, excessive appetite, compulsivity, and some components of depression.

Strategies for Implementing Combination Therapy

Combination treatment can be usefully divided into add-on therapy and co-therapy. In add-on use, drug B is added to drug A, which is already in use. In co-therapy, both drugs are started concurrently. As noted in Chapter 2, the recent published acute mania studies that have shown efficacy of combination therapy regimens have primarily employed add-on designs. The one study that allowed patients to be enrolled with either an add-on use or co-therapy initiation of an antipsychotic plus mood stabilizer at the start of the study found that only the group who had add-on of risperidone to mood stabilizer showed a significantly greater response with the combination regimen (Sachs et al. 2002). As mentioned previously, data regarding combination therapy for maintenance therapy is very limited. Therefore, unless time urgency requires otherwise, current evidence supports addition of a second drug to the first in maintenance therapy rather than concurrent initiation of two drugs. There are insufficient data to recommend a specific duration of trial of a first drug before addition of a second. However, if there is sufficient acuity, concurrently starting a mood stabilizer plus an antipsychotic for mania, or an antidepressant plus a mood stabilizer or atypical antipsychotic for bipolar depression, may be considered. Therefore, clinical necessity is at present the best guide to such decisions.

Similarly, data regarding whether to maintain a combination regimen or taper one of the drugs are also limited. Recent articles addressing this issue have generally reported samples of convenience, where decisions to continue or to stop initially efficacious combination therapy regimens were not made randomly but based on clinical information. Results form such trials may be biased by the treating physicians having started and/or changed regimens based on the clinical state of the particular patient. In general, trial tapering of one of a group of drugs is warranted following a period of relative wellness and stability. If symptoms or illness course worsen, return to combination therapy on a more indefinite basis would be warranted.

Conclusions

Bipolar disorder is a complex, chronic, recurrent lifelong illness that causes tremendous individual suffering and societal costs when untreated or inadequately treated. The recent shift in the focus of treatment from short-term to long-term, from episodic to illness-based, and from syndromal to functional recovery has occurred at least in part as a result of the expansion of long-term treatment options for this illness. Successful outcome in this illness, like in any chronic illness, hinges on applying a holistic approach that encompasses identifying and addressing psychosocial factors impacting compliance; aggressively treating comorbid medical conditions and substance abuse/addiction; and using medications that are effective, safe, and tolerable in the long term. Because bipolar illness is multidimensional, successful management frequently requires skillful combinations of medications and psychosocial interventions.

References

Ahlfors UG, Baastrup PC, Dencker SJ, et al: Flupenthixol decanoate in recurrent manic-depressive illness: a comparison with lithium. Acta Psychiatr Scand 64:226–237, 1981

Altamura AC, Salvadori D, Madaro D, et al: Efficacy and tolerability of quetiapine in the treatment of bipolar disorder: preliminary evidence from a 12-month open-label study. J Affect Disord 76:267–271, 2003

Altshuler LL, Post RM, Leverich GS, et al: Antidepressant-induced mania and cycle acceleration: a controversy revisited. Am J Psychiatry 152:1130–1138, 1995

Altshuler L, Suppes T, Black D, et al: Impact of antidepressant discontinuation after acute bipolar depression remission on rates of depressive relapse at 1-year follow-up. Am J Psychiatry 160:1252–1262, 2003

American Diabetes Association, American Psychiatric Association, American Association of Clinical Endocrinologists, et al: Consensus development conference on antipsychotic drugs and obesity and diabetes. Diabetes Care 27:596–601, 2004

American Psychiatric Association: Practice guideline for the treatment of patients with bipolar disorder (revision). Am J Psychiatry 159(suppl):1–50, 2002

Baldessarini RJ, Tohen M, Tondo L: Maintenance treatment in bipolar disorder. Arch Gen Psychiatry 57:490–492, 2000

Bowden CL, Gonzales CL: Prevention of recurrences in patients with bipolar disorder, in Treatment of Recurrent Depression (Review of Psychiatry, Vol 20). Edited by Greden JF. Washington, DC, American Psychiatric Publishing, 2001, pp 81–101

Bowden CL, Calabrese JR, McElroy SL, et al: A randomized, placebo-controlled 12-month trial of divalproex and lithium in treatment of outpatients with bipolar I disorder. Arch Gen Psychiatry 57:481–489, 2000

Bowden CL, Calabrese JR, Sachs G, et al: A placebo-controlled 18-month trial of lamotrigine and lithium maintenance treatment in recently manic or hypomanic patients with bipolar I disorder. Arch Gen Psychiatry 60:392–400, 2003

Bowden CL, Ketter TA, Calabrese JR, et al: Predictors of response to maintenance treatements with lithium, lamotrigine, and placebo in bipolar disorder patients. Paper presented at the annual meeting of the American Psychiatric Association, Washington, DC, May 2003

Calabrese JR, Shelton MD: Long-term treatment of bipolar disorder with lamotrigine. J Clin Psychiatry 63:18–22, 2002

Calabrese JR, Bowden CL, McElroy SL, et al: Spectrum of activity of lamotrigine in treatment-refractory bipolar disorder. Am J Psychiatry 156:1019–1023, 1999a

Calabrese JR, Bowden CL, Sachs GS, et al: A double-blind placebo-controlled study of lamotrigine monotherapy in outpatients with bipolar I depression. J Clin Psychiatry 60:79–88, 1999b

Calabrese JR, Suppes T, Bowden CL, et al: A double-blind placebo-controlled prophylaxis study of lamotrigine in rapid cycling bipolar disorder. J Clin Psychiatry 61:841–850, 2000

Calabrese JR, Bowden CL, Sachs G, et al: A placebo-controlled 18-month trial of lamotrigine and lithium maintenance treatment in recently depressed patients with bipolar I disorder. J Clin Psychiatry 64:1013–1024, 2003a

Calabrese JR, Vieta E, Shelton MD. Latest maintenance data on lamotrigine in bipolar disorder. Eur Neuropsychopharmacol 13:S57–S66, 2003b

Colom F, Vieta E, Martinez-Aran A, et al: A randomized trial on the efficacy of group psychoeducation in the prophylaxis of recurrences in bipolar patients whose disease is in remission. Arch Gen Psychiatry 60:402–407, 2003a

Colom F, Vieta E, Reinares M, et al: Psychoeducation efficacy in bipolar disorders: beyond compliance enhancement. J Clin Psychiatry 64:1101–1105, 2003b

Coryell W, Winokur G, Solomon D, et al: Lithium and recurrence in a long-term follow-up of bipolar affective disorder. Psychol Med 27:281–289, 1997

DelBello MP, Schwiers ML, Rosenberg HL, et al: A double-blind, randomized, placebo-controlled study of quetiapine as adjunctive treatment for adolescent mania. J Am Acad Child Adolesc Psychiatry 41:1216–1223, 2002

Denicoff KD, Smith-Jackson EE, Disney ER, et al: Comparative prophylactic efficacy of lithium, carbamazepine, and the combination in bipolar disorder. J Clin Psychiatry 58:470–478, 1997

Dunner DL, Stallone F, Fieve RR: Lithium carbonate and affective disorders V: a double-blind study of prophylaxis of depression in bipolar illness. Arch Gen Psychiatry 33:117–120, 1976

Evans DA, Nemeroff CB: The dexamethasone suppression test in mixed bipolar disorder. Am J Psychiatry 140:615–617, 1983

Gelenberg AJ, Kane JM, Keller MB, et al: Comparison of standard and low serum levels of lithium for maintenance treatment of bipolar disorder. N Engl J Med 321:1489–1493, 1989

Gitlin MJ, Swendsen J, Heller TL, et al: Relapse and impairment in bipolar disorder. Am J Psychiatry 152:1635–1640, 1995

Goldberg RJ: Practical Guide to the Care of the Psychiatric Patient. St. Louis, MO, Mosby, 1998

Goodwin FK: Rationale of long-term treatment of bipolar disorder and evidence for long-term lithium treatment. J Clin Psychiatry 63:5–12, 2002

Goodwin FK, Jamison KR: Manic-Depressive Illness. New York, Oxford University Press, 1990

Goodwin GM, Bowden CL, Calabrese JR, et al: A pooled analysis of two placebo-controlled 18-month trials of lamotrigine and lithium maintenance in bipolar I disorder. J Clin Psychiatry 65:432–441, 2004

Greil W, Ludwig-Mayerhofer W, Erazo N, et al: Lithium versus carbamazepine in the maintenance treatment of bipolar disorders: a randomised study. J Affect Disord 43:151–161, 1997

Greil W, Kleindienst N, Erazo N, et al: Differential response to lithium and carbamazepine in the prophylaxis of bipolar disorder. J Clin Psychopharmacol 18:455–460, 1998

Gyulai L, Bowden CL, McElroy SL, et al: Maintenance efficacy of divalproex in the prevention of bipolar depression. Neuropsychopharmacology 28:1374–1382, 2003

Harrow M, Goldberg JF, Grossman LS, et al: Outcome in manic disorders: a naturalistic follow-up study. Arch Gen Psychiatry 47:665–671, 1990

Hartong EG, Moleman P, Hoogduin CA, et al: Prophylactic efficacy of lithium versus carbamazepine in treatment-naive bipolar patients. J Clin Psychiatry 64:144–151, 2003

Hlastala SA, Frank E, Mallinger AG, et al: Bipolar depression: an underestimated treatment challenge. Depress Anxiety 5:73–83, 1997

Horgan D: Change of diagnosis to manic depressive illness. Psychol Med 11:517–523, 1981

Jackson A, Cavanagh J, Scott J: A systematic review of prodromal symptoms of mania and depression. J Affect Disord 74:209–217; 2003

Jacobsen FM: Low dose valproate: a new treatment for cyclothymia, mild rapid cycling disorders, and premenstrual syndrome. J Clin Psychiatry 54:229–234, 1993

Johnson RE, McFarland BH: Lithium use and discontinuation in a health maintenance organization. Am J Psychiatry 153:993–1000, 1996

Keck PE, Meinhold JM, Prihoda TJ, et al: Relation of serum valproate and lithium concentrations to efficacy and tolerability in maintenance therapy for bipolar disorder. Paper presented at the annual meeting of the American College of Neuropsychopharmacology, San Juan, Puerto Rico, December 2002

Keck PE Jr, Potkin SG, Giller E Jr, et al: Ziprasidone's long-term efficacy and safety in bipolar disorder. Presented at the 157th annual meeting of the American Psychiatric Association, New York, May 2004a

Keck PE Jr, Sanchez R, Marcus RN, et al: Aripiprazole for relapse prevention in bipolar disorder in a 26-week trial. Presented at the 157th annual meeting of the American Psychiatric Association, New York, May 2004b

Ketter TA, Tohen MF, Vieta E, et al: Open-label maintenance treatment for bipolar depression using olanzapine or olanzapine/fluoxetine combination: International Society for Bipolar Disorders Regional Group Conference, Sydney, Australia, February 5–7 2004 (abstract 309). Bipolar Disord 6 (suppl 1):27, 2004

Krishnan RR, Maltbie AA, Davidson JR: Abnormal cortisol suppression in bipolar patients with simultaneous manic and depressive symptoms. Am J Psychiatry 140:203–205, 1983

Kusumakar V: Antidepressant and antipsychotics in the long term treatment of bipolar disorder. J Clin Psychiatry 63:23–28, 2002

Lam DH, Watkins ER, Hayward P, et al: A randomized controlled study of cognitive therapy for relapse prevention for bipolar affective disorder. Arch Gen Psychiatry 60:145–152; 2003

Lambert PA, Venaud G: Comparative study of valpromide versus lithium as prophylactic treatment in affective disorders. Nervure 5:57–65, 1992

Levine J, Chengappa KN, Brar JS, et al: Psychotropic drug prescription patterns among patients with bipolar I disorder. Bipolar Disord 2:120–130, 2000

Maj M, Pirozzi R, Magliano L, et al: Long-term outcome of lithium prophylaxis in bipolar disorder: a 5-year prospective study of 402 patients at a lithium clinic. Am J Psychiatry 155:30–35, 1998

Martinez-Aran A, Vieta E, Reinares M, et al: Cognitive function across manic or hypomanic, depressed, and euthymic states in bipolar disorder. Am J Psychiatry 161:262–270, 2004

Metz A, Bowden C, Calabrese J, et al: Concomitant use of lamotrigine and valproate in bipolar I disorder. Abstract presented at the American College of Neuropsychopharmacology Annual Meeting, San Juan, Puerto Rico, December 2002

Miklowitz DJ, Goldstein MJ: Behavioral family treatment for patients with bipolar affective disorder. Behav Modif 14:457–489, 1990

Miklowitz DJ, Simoneau TL, George EL, et al: Family-focused treatment of bipolar disorder: 1-year effects of a psychoeducational program in conjuction with pharmacotherapy. Biol Psychiatry 48:582–592; 2000

Miklowitz DJ, George EL, Richards JA, et al: A randomized study of family focused psychoeducation and pharmacotherapy in the outpatient management of bipolar disorder. Arch Gen Psychiatry 60:904–912, 2003

Moncrieff J: Lithium revisited. A re-examination of the placebo-controlled trials of lithium prophylaxis in manic-depressive disorder (editorial). Br J Psychiatry 167:569–573, 1995

Muller-Oerlinghausen B, Retzow A, Henn FA, et al: Valproate as an adjunct to neuroleptic medication for the treatment of acute episodes of mania: a prospective, randomized, double-blind, placebo-controlled, multicenter study. J Clin Psychopharmacol 20:195–203, 2000

Perlis RH, Sachs GS, Lafer B, et al: Effect of abrupt change from standard to low serum level so lithium: a reanalysis of double-blind lithium maintenance data. Am J Psychiatry 159:1155–1159, 2004

Perry A, Terrier N, Morriss R, et al: Randomized controlled clinical trail of efficacy of teaching patients with bipolar disorder to identify early symptoms of relapse and obtain treatment. BMJ 318:149–153, 1999

Post RM, Denicoff KD, Frye MA, et al: Re-evaluating carbamazepine prophylaxis in bipolar disorder. Br J Psychiatry 170:202–204, 1997

Revicki DA, Paramore LC, Sommerville KW, et al: Divalproex sodium versus olanzapine in the treatment of bipolar disorder: health related quality of life and medical cost outcomes. J Clin Psychiatry 64:288–294, 2003

Sachs G, Grossman F, Okamoto A, et al: Risperidone plus mood stabilizer versus placebo plus mood stabilizer for acute mania of bipolar disorder: a double-blind comparison of efficacy and safety. Am J Psychiatry 159:1146–1154, 2002

Scott J, Pope M: Nonadherence with mood stabilizers: prevalence and predictors. J Clin Psychiatry 63:384–390, 2002

Silverstone T, Romans S, Hunt N, et al: Is there a seasonal pattern of relapse in bipolar affective disorders? A dual northern and southern hemisphere cohort study. Br J Psychiatry 167:58–60, 1995

Solomon DA, Ryan CE, Keitner GI, et al: A pilot study of lithium carbonate plus divalproex sodium for the continuation and maintenance treatment of patients with bipolar I disorder. J Clin Psychiatry 58:95–99, 1997

Suppes T, Webb A, Paul B, et al: Clinical outcome in a randomized 1-year trial of clozapine versus treatment as usual for patients with treatment-resistant illness and a history of mania. Am J Psychiatry 156:1164–1169, 1999

Suppes T, McElroy SL, Keck PE, et al: Use of quetiapine in bipolar disorder: a case series with prospective evaluation. Int Clin Psychopharmacol 19:173–174, 2004

Swann AC, Secunda SK, Stokes PE, et al: Stress, depression, and mania: relationship between perceived role of stressful events and clinical and biochemical characteristics. Acta Psychiatr Scand 81:389–397, 1990

Swann AC, Bowden CL, Calabrese JR, et al: Differential effect of number of previous episodes of affective disorder on response to lithium or divalproex in acute mania. Am J Psychiatry 156:1264–1266, 1999

Swann AC, Janicak PL, Calabrese JR, et al: Structure of mania: depressive, irritable, and psychotic clusters with distinct course of illness in randomized clinical trial participants. J Affect Disord 67:123–132, 2001

Swann AC, Bowden CL, Calabrese JR, et al: Pattern of response to divalproex, lithium, or placebo in four naturalistic subtypes of mania. Neuropsychopharmacology 26:530–536, 2002

Tohen M, Hennen J, Zarate CM Jr, et al: Two-year syndromal and functional recovery in 219 cases of first-episode major affective disorder with psychotic features. Am J Psychiatry 157:220–228, 2000

Tohen M, Chengappa KNR, Suppes T, et al: Efficacy of olanzapine in combination with valproate or lithium in the treatment of mania in patients partially nonresponsive to valproate or lithium monotherapy. Arch Gen Psychiatry 59:62–69, 2002

Tohen MF, Bowden CL, Calabrese JR, et al: Olanzapine versus placebo for relapse prevention in bipolar disorder. Presented at the 156th annual meeting of the American Psychiatric Association, San Francisco, CA, May 2003a

Tohen M, Ketter TA, Zarate CA, et al: Olanzapine versus divalproex sodium for the treatment of acute mania and maintenance of remission: a 47-week study. Am J Psychiatry 160:1263–1271, 2003b

Tohen MF, Marneros A, Bowden CL, et al: Olanzapine versus lithium in relapse prevention in bipolar disorder. Presented at the 156th annual meeting of the American Psychiatric Association, San Francisco, CA, May 2003c

Tohen M, Chengappa KN, Suppes T, et al: Relapse prevention in bipolar I disorder: 18-month comparison of olanzapine plus mood stabiliser v. mood stabiliser alone. Br J Psychiatry 184:337–345, 2004

Vestergaard P, Licht RW, Brodersen A, et al: Outcome of lithium pro-phylaxis: a prospective follow-up of affective disorder patients as-signed to high and low serum lithium levels. Acta Psychiatr Scand 98:310–315, 1998

Vieta E, Goikolea JM, Corbella B, et al: Risperidone safety and efficacy in the treatment of bipolar and schizoaffective disorders: results from a 6-month, multicenter, open study. J Clin Psychiatry 62:818–825, 2001

Weisler RH, Warrington L, Dunn J, et al: Adjunctive ziprasidone in bi-polar mania: short-term and long-term data. Presented at the 157th annual meeting of the American Psychiatric Association, New York, May 2004

Yatham LN, Grossman F, Augustyns I, et al: Mood stabilisers plus ris-peridone or placebo in the treatment of acute mania: international, double-blind, randomised controlled trial. Br J Psychiatry 182:141–147, 2003

Yatham LN, Paulsson B, Mullen J, et al: Quetiapine versus placebo in combination with lithium or divalproex for the treatment of bipolar mania. J Clin Psychopharmacol 24599–606, 2004

Chapter 5

Treatment of Rapid-Cycling Bipolar Disorder

David J. Muzina, M.D.
Omar Elhaj, M.D.
Prashant Gajwani, M.D.
Keming Gao, M.D., Ph.D.
Joseph R. Calabrese, M.D.

In 1913, Emil Kraepelin originally described what likely became *rapid-cycling bipolar disorder* as "manic-depressive insanity" (Kraepelin 1913). Kraepelin distinguished manic-depressive illness from the degenerative course of schizophrenia by its periodic cycling and noted that cycling occurred with remarkable frequency in a subgroup of patients with bipolar disorder. Dunner and Fieve (1974) coined the term *rapid cycling* many years later while describing clinical factors associated with lithium prophylaxis failure in bipolar disorder. Rapid cycling was used to describe the occurrence of four or more mood episodes per year, with the typical course of mania or hypomania followed by depression. Several studies confirmed the validity of rapid cycling as a distinct course specifier for bipolar disorder, most notably a meta-analysis completed by Bauer et al. (1994), which led to its inclusion in DSM-IV (American Psychiatric Association 1994) and now DSM-IV-TR (American Psychiatric Association 2000).

According to DSM-IV-TR, the course specifier of rapid cycling applies to "at least four episodes of a mood disturbance in the previous 12 months that meet criteria for a Major Depressive, Manic, Mixed, or Hypomanic Episode" (American Psychiatric Association 2000, p. 428). The episodes must be "demarcated either by partial or full remission for at least 2 months or a switch to an episode of opposite polarity" (p. 428). Alternative definitions of rapid cycling have been proposed, usually suggesting consideration of recurrent affective episodes that do not always meet the duration or remission criteria set forth by DSM-IV-TR for each individual episode. Early studies often employed these alternative rapid cycling definitions, suggesting that the DSM-IV and DSM-IV-TR criteria cover only part of a spectrum of rapid cycling conditions (Maj et al. 1999).

The prevalence rate of rapid cycling in bipolar disorder is estimated to range from 13% to 56% (Akiskal et al. 2000; Angst and Sellaro 2000), frequently presenting late in the course of illness and occurring more commonly in women (as discussed by Rasgon and Zappert in Chapter 7) and in those patients with bipolar type II disorder. Rapid cycling is seen almost exclusively in bipolar disorder, rarely in unipolar depression, and is associated with greater short- and long-term morbidity, presenting more difficult treatment challenges for clinicians. Indeed, growing interest in the concept of rapid cycling has corresponded with observations that patients with rapid-cycling bipolar disorder did not respond adequately when treated with lithium and that other medications, such as divalproex sodium, were more effective particularly for the hypomanic or manic phases of the illness (Calabrese and Delucchi 1990; Dunner and Fieve 1974; Kukopulos et al. 1980). Recent reports challenge the assertion that lithium is less effective than divalproex for rapid-cycling bipolar disorder (Calabrese et al., in press). Evidence from follow-up studies suggests that rapid cycling is more representative of a severe phase of bipolar illness rather than a distinct subtype (Maj et al. 1994).

Rapid cycling causes considerable distress and suffering, particularly owing to the frequent recurrence of treatment-refractory depression that has been described as the hallmark of the illness (Calabrese et al. 2001a). Antidepressant use may exacerbate or destabilize the course of rapid-cycling bipolar disorder through cycle induction or acceleration, further adding to the challenge of treating these affectively fragile patients.

Appropriate selection of a mood-stabilizing regimen is increasingly important for the management of bipolar illness when a rapid-cycling pattern emerges. Consensus expert opinion recommends that foundational treatment of rapid-cycling bipolar disorder should consist of initial treatment with first-line mood stabilizers such as lithium, divalproex, or lamotrigine. Choosing initial therapy is challenging given the absence of consistent data to guide clinical practice. When rapid cycling appears in a previously stable bipolar patient on maintenance therapy, further mood stabilization through optimization of medication dosing or combination therapies becomes clearly necessary. This is particularly germane because available data suggest that current monotherapy strategies are generally inadequate to treat this difficult variant of bipolar illness and that an individually tailored medication regimen consisting of two or more agents may be the best strategy for effective treatment in both the acute and maintenance phases. In general, antidepressants should be avoided because of the increased potential for acceleration of mood swings or induction of mania. Controlled trials in homogeneous cohorts of patients with rapid-cycling bipolar disorder are still needed to better illuminate the best pharmacological treatment strategies for breaking the rapid-cycling phase and providing better long-term mood stability.

The objective of this chapter is to review the available literature on the advancing treatments of rapid-cycling bipolar disorder with an emphasis on evidence-based recommendations from controlled trials. We focus on the use of lithium, divalproex, carbamazepine, olanzapine, lamotrigine, and quetiapine.

Lithium

Evidence

Early observations led to the conclusion that lithium was ineffective in the treatment of rapid-cycling bipolar disorder. Some clinicians have additionally argued that lithium has poor efficacy in treating rapid-cycling bipolar disorder even when supplemented by antidepressants and neuroleptics (Bowden 2001; Post et al. 2000). In contrast, other reports have supported lithium efficacy in the treatment of rapid-cycling bipolar disorder (Baldessarini et al. 2002; Tondo et al. 2001; Viguera et al. 2001).

In an attempt to clarify factors associated with the failure of lithium prophylaxis in all types of bipolar disorder, Dunner and Fieve (1974) carried out a placebo-controlled, double-blind maintenance study in a general cohort of 55 patients, of whom 20% were rapid cyclers. A disproportionate number of rapid cyclers were represented in the lithium failure group, with 82% (9 of 11) of rapid cyclers failing lithium therapy compared with 41% (18 of 44) of non–rapid cyclers. This led to the conclusion that lithium did not work well for rapid cycling. Lithium failure was defined in this study as hospitalization for, or treatment of, mania or depression during lithium therapy or mood symptoms as documented by rating scales sufficient to warrant a diagnosis of mild depression or hypomania/mania persisting for at least 2 weeks. However, although the majority of patients with rapid cycling continued to be ill after more than 2 years of lithium therapy, the time spent in remission increased over 3 years of study. One year of lithium therapy led to an average of 8 months of euthymia, mainly by decreasing the time patients spent either hypomanic or manic.

Kukopulos (1980) replicated the findings of Dunner and Fieve in a study of the longitudinal clinical course of 434 bipolar patients. Fifty of these patients were rapid cyclers on continuous lithium therapy for more than 1 year, with poor response in 72% and good-to-partial prophylaxis in only 28%. However, the allowance of concomitant antidepressant medications for intervening depressive episodes may have confounded these results. Maj et al. (1998) later published a 5-year prospective study of lithium therapy in a general cohort of 402 patients with bipolar disorder and noted the absence of rapid cycling in good responders to lithium but an incidence rate of 26% in nonresponders to lithium.

Baldessarini et al. (2000) concluded that rapid-cycling bipolar disorder was strongly associated with bipolar type II diagnosis, higher average pre-lithium episode frequency and percentage of time ill, and weakly associated with the female sex but not with greater overall morbidity during treatment. In 360 subjects with DSM-IV bipolar I (n=218) or II (n=142) disorder (64% women) followed over an average of 13.3 years, researchers used bivariate and multivariate techniques to evaluate factors associated with rapid-cycling status and response to lithium maintenance treatment (recurrence rates, time ill, survival analysis of time to recurrence on lithium). Their results indicated that the risk for rapid cycling (15.6%) was 5.1 times greater in subjects with bipolar II versus bipolar I disorder (30.3% versus 6.0%); in minor excess in women versus men (17.9% versus 11.5%); and associated with premorbid cyclothymia, depressive first episodes, older age of onset, and being employed or married. Before lithium, rapid-cycling versus non–rapid-cycling cases had higher mean total number of manic and depressive episodes per year (3.9 versus 1.2) and greater percentage of time ill (60% versus 38%). During treatment, prior rapid-cycling status was unrelated to time to first recurrence and other measures of morbidity and improvement, including time ill, although depressive episodes were 2.7 times more frequent, and there was 13.7% less chance of full protection from all recurrences in rapid-cycling cases. Limitations of this study included its naturalistic design and the lack of random assignment or blind assessment.

Previous depressive and manic episodes may have a differential effect on response to treatment with lithium (Swann et al. 2000). For predictive factors, 179 subjects in three parallel groups (divalproex, lithium, placebo) were evaluated over a period of 21 days using structured interviews conducted by the clinician (Schedule for Affective Disorders and Schizophrenia–Change [SADS-C]) and by nursing staff (Affective Disorders Rating Scale [ADRS]). For the follow-up study, 372 stabilized patients were randomized to three groups: divalproex, lithium, or placebo. Observations from this study led to the conclusion that a history of at least 4 previous depressive or 12 previous manic episodes is associated with reduced antimanic response to lithium. Response to lithium, but not to divalproex or placebo, worsened with increased depressive or manic episodes. Having more than 11 manic or 4 depressive episodes was associated with response to lithium that did not differ from placebo. Effects of previous depressive and manic episodes appeared independent and could not be accounted for by increased rapid cycling or mixed states. There was a tendency for subjects with four or more previous depressive episodes to be women (25 of 57 versus only 20 women of 70 subjects with three or fewer episodes, $\chi^2=3.2$, $P=0.07$). Although subjects with many episodes had a high incidence of rapid cycling, only one subject with more than 11 manic episodes randomized to lithium had rapid cycling. Therefore, the reduced response to lithium occurred among subjects who were not rapid cyclers, and current rapid cycling did not account for the reduced response to lithium in patients with many previous episodes of mania or of depression. This cross-sectional dataset cannot distinguish whether this phenomenon represents progressive development of lithium resistance with repeated episodes or indicates that those patients who had frequent episodes were also lithium resistant from the start. The reported increased episodes could be associated with increased incidents of lithium discontinuation, which may have led to neurophysiological changes adversely affecting response to lithium but not to divalproex. However, previous favorable response to lithium in the present study predicted favorable response in the index episode, arguing against loss of lithium response with repeated episodes of treatment. Furthermore, most patients had similar responsiveness to lithium before and after lithium discontinuation.

Viguera et al. (2001) compared the clinical characteristics of 360 women and men with DSM-IV bipolar I or II disorder before and during lithium maintenance monotherapy. Using preliminary bivariate comparisons, multivariate analysis, and survival analysis of time stable during treatment, they found that women were 1.6 times more likely than men to have type II disorder, were 3.2 years older at illness onset, were depressed 1.4 times more often, considered to be unipolar depressive 1.9 years longer, and started maintenance treatment 5.5 years later. However, women differed little from men before treatment in overall morbidity, average episode frequency, and risk of suicide attempts. Women showed nonsignificantly superior responses to lithium treatment and a significant 60% longer median time before a first recurrence during treatment, despite 7% lower average serum lithium concentrations. Women were diagnosed as having bipolar disorder later than men, with corresponding delay of lithium maintenance treatment that proved to be at least as effective as in men.

Other reports suggest a more favorable response to lithium in patients with rapid cycling. This may be particularly true for bipolar type II patients and those not treated with antidepressants. In a select cohort of lithium-responsive patients with bipolar I or II disorder, Tondo et al. (1998) concluded that lithium maintenance generates significant long-term reductions in depressive as well as manic morbidity, particularly in the type II subset. In some patients with rapid cycling, simply discontinuing antidepressant drugs may allow lithium to act as a more effective anticycling mood-stabilizing agent (Wehr et al. 1988). Notably, at least eight placebo-controlled, randomized trials have shown lithium to have prophylactic efficacy in bipolar disorder (Goodwin 2002). Along with results from a meta-analysis of 16 studies of bipolar disorder prophylaxis exposing no evidence for differing efficacy in rapid cycling among the mood stabilizers (Tondo et al. 2003), the current body of evidence in totality suggests consideration of lithium for first-line prophylaxis of bipolar disorder, with or without rapid cycling.

Practical Considerations

Lithium is contraindicated in patients with severe cardiovascular or renal disease and in those with evidence of severe debilitation or dehydration or with sodium depletion. Mild to moderate adverse effects may occur even when plasma lithium levels are below 1 mEq/L. Rapid rises in serum lithium concentrations may result in post-absorptive symptoms associated with the most frequent adverse effects during lithium initiation: nausea and other gastrointestinal disturbances, vertigo, and muscle weakness. These effects frequently disappear after stabilization of therapy. The more common and persistent adverse effects include fine tremor of the hands, fatigue, polydipsia/polyuria, and nephrogenic diabetes insipidus. Toxic reactions may occur at lithium concentrations of 1.5–2 mEq/L and more severe reactions at concentrations greater than 2 mEq/L.

Some patients may experience lithium accumulation during initial therapy, increasing to toxic concentrations and requiring immediate discontinuation of the drug. Elderly patients or those with lower renal clearances for lithium may also be at increased risk for toxicity, requiring reduction or temporary discontinuation of lithium. Otherwise, in the absence of renal excretion problems, toxic manifestations of lithium become visible in a predictable sequence related to serum lithium concentrations. The usually transient gastrointestinal symptoms are the earliest side effects to occur and tremor may emerge or worsen. Early intoxication may be heralded by polyuria and polydipsia, followed by increased drowsiness, ataxia, tinnitus, and blurring of vision. The progressive signs of lithium toxicity may then quickly manifest with confusion or frank disorientation, muscle fasciculations or twitching, hyperreflexia, nystagmus, seizures, diarrhea, vomiting, and eventually coma and death.

The initial clinical response to the appearance of inadequate lithium response should be to review the patient's adherence to the medication regimen and to ensure optimal dosing and duration of treatment. Often, patients may become poorly compliant with lithium therapy due to the emergence of undesirable side effects such as tremor or gastrointestinal disturbances. Lithium-induced tremor may be alleviated by relatively low dosages of beta-blockers (e.g., propranolol 20 mg three times daily). Gastrointestinal disturbances can be reduced by switching lithium preparations, with change to slow-release lithium helpful for nausea and conversion to immediate-release lithium often resolving diarrhea. Thyroid supplementation may improve the cognitive slowing that many lithium-treated patients report, with or without laboratory evidence for hypothyroidism (Tremont and Stern 1997).

Although reducing the dosage of lithium may decrease these dose-dependent side effects, doing so may also substantially attenuate its prophylactic powers. The ideal lithium serum level for optimum mood stabilization may indeed require individual tailoring on a case-by-case basis; however, available evidence should guide these efforts. There is an incremental side effect burden with rising lithium levels but greater efficacy at the higher end of lithium's therapeutic serum level range (Maj et al. 1986). A reasonable minimum target level in the 0.61–0.75 mEq/L range may offer the best balance between efficacy and side effects.

The duration of time treated with lithium is also an important practical consideration when determining efficacy. Benefits may not manifest for 6 months or longer as evidenced by a comparison of bipolar patients randomized to lithium versus carbamazepine that showed gradual decrease in interepisode morbidity over the first 6 months of lithium treatment, but not carbamazepine therapy, followed by stabilization for the remaining 2.5 years of observation (Kleindienst and Greil 2002).

Divalproex

Evidence

As with lithium, the evidence for divalproex from mostly open studies of rapid-cycling bipolar disorder suggests a moderate to marked efficacy in manic and mixed phases but poor to moderate efficacy in the depressed phase. Divalproex also appears better able to prevent future manic or mixed episodes than depressive relapses in rapidly cycling bipolar patients.

A prospective, open label study of divalproex in patients with lithium-refractory rapid-cycling bipolar disorder found a favorable acute response to divalproex in 54% of manic patients, 87% of patients in a mixed state, and 19% of patients with depressive episodes (Calabrese et al. 1992). Over this study's nearly 16 months of prophylactic treatment on divalproex, marked therapeutic effects were reported for mania in 72% of the sample, 94% for mixed states, and 33% for depression. An open trial of a homogenous cohort of patients with rapid-cycling bipolar disorder found divalproex to possess moderate to marked acute and prophylactic antimanic properties with only modest antidepressant effects (Calabrese and Delucchi 1990). A positive family history of affective disorder, no prior lithium therapy, and bipolar II or mixed states were predictive of a positive response to divalproex, whereas those with more frequent or severe mania or borderline personality disorder were more likely not to respond to divalproex (Calabrese et al. 1992).

Swann (2001) analyzed the prediction pattern of treatment response in acute mania in a controlled clinical trial with divalproex. Over a period of 21 days, 179 subjects in three parallel groups (divalproex, lithium, and placebo) were evaluated using structured interviews conducted by the clinician (SADS-C) and by nursing staff (ADRS). In a follow-up study, 372 stabilized patients were randomized to three groups: divalproex, lithium, or placebo. The results showed that patients with manic episodes with depressive symptoms or with rapid cycling exhibited good response to divalproex. They concluded that high numbers of prior manic and depressive episodes are predictive of poor response to lithium and favorable response to divalproex.

In a 20-month double-blind, maintenance trial of lithium versus divalproex monotherapy in bipolar I and II disorder accompanied by a recent history of rapid cycling, the hypothesis that rapid cycling was a predictor of positive response to divalproex and negative response to lithium was tested (Calabrese et al., submitted for publication). There were no significant differences in time to relapse with either lithium or divalproex. The rate of relapse into any mood episode was 56% on lithium and 51% on divalproex. The rate of relapse into hypomania/mania was 22% for both groups, with a higher relapse into depression for both lithium (34%) and divalproex (29%). These data do not support the previously held notion that divalproex is more effective than lithium in the long-term management of rapid-cycling bipolar disorder.

Combining divalproex with lithium therapy may improve overall response rates (Calabrese et al. 2001a,b; Sharma et al. 1993). Despite this, recurrent depressive episodes remain problematic for many rapid-cycling bipolar patients. In a large cohort of rapid cyclers, including those with comorbid alcohol, cocaine, and/or cannabis abuse, the combined use of lithium and divalproex over 6 months resulted in mood stabilization in less than half of the patients, independent of comorbid substance abuse. Lack of adherence to treatment, not comorbid substance abuse itself, was associated with poorer outcome. The majority (75%) of the non-responders to this combination therapy had treatment-refractory depression (Calabrese et al. 2001a,b), suggesting that even the combination of divalproex and lithium does not possess robust effectiveness for the treatment of depression in the context of rapid cycling, although there is efficacy for this combination in mania and hypomania.

Practical Considerations

Although there is little overall evidence to clearly support the use of divalproex over lithium in rapid cyclers, its use alone or in combination with lithium may benefit patients with a mania-dominant form of rapid-cycling bipolar I disorder or those with moderate to severe cases of rapid cycling. In addition, intolerance to or lack of efficacy with lithium should promptly lead to consideration of divalproex treatment.

Divalproex is contraindicated in patients with significant hepatic disease or dysfunction or known hypersensitivity to the drug. The most commonly reported side effects are nausea, vomiting, and indigestion. At initiation of therapy, these effects typically appear early in the course, are usually transient, and rarely require discontinuation of divalproex. Diarrhea, abdominal cramps, and constipation have also been reported. Although variable effects on appetite and weight have been reported, an increase in appetite and weight gain are more common. Sedation is more commonly reported in patients receiving combination therapy. Hair loss has been observed and is often of concern to patients, but this effect is most often transient and does not cause gross alopecia. As discussed in Chapter 7, the risks of teratogenicity and polycystic ovarian syndrome need to be considered in women of reproductive age. Skin rash, photosensitivity, petechiae, Stevens-Johnson syndrome, irregular menses, secondary amenorrhea, breast enlargement, galactorrhea, and parotid gland swelling have rarely been reported. In short-term, placebo-controlled trials with bipolar patients, the most commonly reported adverse events were nausea, headache, somnolence, pain, vomiting, and dizziness. In the long-term bipolar studies, the most commonly reported adverse events were somnolence, tremor, headache, asthenia, diarrhea, and nausea.

Carbamazepine

Evidence

Early reports suggested rapid cycling was a predictor of positive response to carbamazepine—the first anticonvulsant investigated as a treatment for bipolar disorder (Post et al. 1987). However, the paucity of controlled studies of carbamazepine prospectively evaluated in a homogeneous cohort of rapid cyclers challenges this early finding. In addition, Okuma (1993) reported that a recent or remote history of rapid cycling predicted a limited response to either carbamazepine or lithium. This study was later supported by a 3-year crossover study of 31 patients with bipolar disorder treated with either lithium or carbamazepine for the first year, switched to the other agent for the second year, and then placed on the combination of lithium and carbamazepine during the third year (Denicoff et al. 1997). Among rapid-cycling patients, only a 19% response rate was reported for the carbamazepine-treated group, compared with a 28% response rate among the lithium-treated group and a much higher combination therapy response rate of 56%. A beneficial effect with this combination therapy had previously been reported, with earlier improvement noted when carbamazepine was co-administered with lithium (Di Costanzo and Schifano 1991; Joffe 1991).

Limited existing data therefore suggest a limited role for carbamazepine in rapid-cycling bipolar disorder, particularly as a monotherapy. If any effectiveness in clinical treatment is expected with carbamazepine, expert recommendations and experience suggest that this anticonvulsant possesses moderate to marked efficacy in the manic phase and poor to moderate efficacy in the depressed phase of the illness (Calabrese et al. 1994). Addition of carbamazepine to or in combination with another mood stabilizer, particularly lithium, likely offers greater acute and prophylactic advantages than monotherapy. The limitations and potential toxicities of carbamazepine therapy are well known, which has led to increased use of oxcarbazepine—a congener of carbamazepine. Although oxcarbazepine lacks the usual risks and discomforts associated with carbamazepine efficacy, data are not available to confidently recommend this agent in rapid-cycling bipolar disorder.

Practical Considerations

Carbamazepine should not be administered to patients with a history of hepatic disease, acute intermittent porphyria, or serious blood disorders. The most frequently reported side effects with carbamazepine are central nervous system (CNS) related (e.g., headache, sedation/drowsiness, dizziness, diplopia, ataxia), gastrointestinal disturbances (nausea, vomiting), and allergic skin reactions. These usually occur only during the initial phase of therapy, if the initial dosage is too high or rapidly increased, or in elderly patients. Low initial dosing and gradual upward titration can minimize these reactions. CNS adverse reactions may emerge at high dosages, in overdose, or with significant fluctuations in plasma levels, requiring more frequent plasma level monitoring, decreased total daily dosage or dividing it into three or four fractional doses, and occasionally discontinuation of carbamazepine. Hematological, hepatic, cardiovascular, and dermatological reactions are more serious adverse reactions and usually require discontinuation of carbamazepine therapy. In selected patients, carbamazepine's minimal effect on weight may make it an attractive option.

Lamotrigine

Evidence

The consensus from increasing numbers of reports evaluating lamotrigine in bipolar patients suggests that in addition to possessing prophylactic efficacy (as described in Chapter 4), it appears to be effective in rapid cycling. Although it is not effective in the manic phase, lamotrigine appears effective in acute bipolar depression, as described in Chapter 3. This profile complements that of lithium and divalproex.

In a 48-week prospective comparison of open-label lamotrigine as add-on or monotherapy in 41 rapid cyclers and 34 non–rapid cyclers, patients with more severe symptoms of mania did not improve from baseline to last visit. However, subgroups of rapid-cycling patients with both depressive and hypomanic symptoms did significantly improve (Bowden et al. 1999; Calabrese et al. 1999).

Another open label investigation of 14 patients with rapid-cycling bipolar disorder treated with either lithium or lamotrigine as a mood stabilizer found that 57% (4/7) of lithium-treated patients had four or more mood episodes during the 1-year period studied, whereas only 14% (1/7) of lamotrigine-treated patients exhibited the same rapid-cycling course (Walden et al. 2000). Forty-three percent (3/7) of the lamotrigine group experienced no further mood episodes in the year following. There was no evidence of preferential antidepressant or antimanic efficacy. This study is limited by small sample size and open-label design.

A double-blind, placebo-controlled study of patients with refractory mood disorders, including those with rapid cycling, that used a crossover series of three 6-week monotherapy evaluations of lamotrigine, gabapentin, and placebo showed marked antidepressant response in 45% of lamotrigine-treated patients compared with 19% in the placebo group (Frye et al. 2000). Gabapentin did not separate from placebo. The demographic profile of the study participants evaluated in all three treatment phases (N=31) included 18 women and 13 men; 11 with bipolar I and 14 with bipolar II; 23 with rapid cycling and 2 non–rapid cycling; and 6 unipolar patients. This study utilized a randomized, double-blind, crossover design in which patients received gabapentin monotherapy, lamotrigine monotherapy, or placebo for 6 weeks, with two subsequent crossover trials. A 1-week crossover period was implemented between phases. Patients were treated only with the study medications except for the following: four patients who continued receiving stable levothyroxine supplementation for corrected primary hypothyroidism; one patient who continued receiving diuretic therapy for essential hypertension; and two patients, each of whom continued receiving stable prior medications (i.e., triiodothyronine and clonazepam). Lamotrigine was started at a dosage of 25 mg daily for the first week before titration up to 300 to 500 mg daily in the fifth through sixth weeks. The titration schedule was more rapid than that in the current prescribing information. The currect slower approach is necessary to limit the risk of rash. The initial gabapentin dosage was 900 mg/day, titrated to 4,800 mg/day by the fifth through sixth weeks. After completion of all three phases of the study, patients who had responded to a particular phase (I, II, or III) were offered the option of returning to that phase, still on a blinded basis, for response confirmation.

The primary outcome measure of overall improvement was the Clinical Global Impression Scale for Bipolar Disorder (CGI-BP). Supplementary ratings used in the evaluation and completion of the CGI-BP response rating included prospective self- and observer-rated life charting, Hamilton Depression Inventory, Young Mania Rating Scale (YMRS), Spielberger State Anxiety Scale, and Brief Psychiatric Rating Scale. CGI-BP change determinations were made by a consensus of blinded research physicians and clinicians in comparison with both the previous phase of illness and the worst phase of documented illness. Prior treatment exposure and documented treatment failures, including therapeutic level with inadequate response, clinical intolerance, or affective relapse, were the following: for lithium, 28 of 31 (90%) patients experienced prior exposure and 28 of 28 (100%) patients experienced prior treatment failure; for valproic acid, 26 of 31 (84%) and 21 of 26 (81%), respectively; and for carbamazepine, 20 of 31 (65%) and 14 of 20 (70%), respectively.

For those patients who completed all three phases, Cochran's Q statistic was used to compare overall CGI-BP response with any significant statistic followed by a post hoc test. This allowed pairwise comparisons of the proportion of responders in the medication phases to determine the location of a difference. The Fisher exact test was used for differential response rates based on gender status.

The mean daily dosages at week 6 were 274 ± 128 mg for lamotrigine and $3,987 \pm 856$ mg for gabapentin. There was no difference in lamotrigine and gabapentin doses between responders and nonresponders. The response rates based on the overall CGI-BP rating of much or very much improved were the following: lamotrigine, 52% (16/31); gabapentin, 26% (8/31), and placebo, 23% (7/31). Post hoc Q differences ($df=1$, $N=31$) were the following: lamotrigine versus gabapentin ($Q_{diff}=5.33$, $P=0.011$); lamotrigine versus placebo ($Q_{diff}=4.76$, $P=0.022$); and gabapentin versus placebo ($Q_{diff}=0.08$, $P=0.700$). Only a trend level of significance was reached for the CGI-BP response rates for separate manic and depressive components of the illness. The response rates for mania were the following: lamotrigine, 44% (11/25); gabapentin, 20% (5/25); and placebo, 32% (8/25). For depression, the response rates were the following: lamotrigine, 45% (14/31);

gabapentin, 26% (8/31); and placebo, 19% (6/31). The response rate observed during just phase I was highly similar to that for the whole study using all three phases of the crossover trial: 50% (5/10) for lamotrigine, 33% (3/9) for gabapentin, and 18% (2/11) for placebo. In addition, when the response data were analyzed as a function of a positive response in the preceding phase, only 23% of lamotrigine responders, 50% of gabapentin responders, and 0% of placebo responders were also partial responders in the previous phase and would thus have entered the next phase somewhat improved. This finding further indicates that there were not a greater percentage of lamotrigine-responsive patients who were responders in the preceding phase. Moreover, there were no significant differences at the baseline level on any of the supplementary ratings of severity of illness. There was no difference between the response rates based on gender. Both agents were generally well tolerated, with the exception of one patient, who was administered lamotrigine and developed a rash after the 6-week study phase was over; this rash occurred in week 15 (during the continuation treatment), progressed to toxic epidermal necrolysis, and required the patient to be hospitalized in an intensive care burn unit. The patient recovered fully. This case emphasizes the importance of using the current slower titration schedule for lamotrigine in efforts to limit the risk of serious rash. A pairwise contrast (lamotrigine versus gabapentin, $F=5.884$, $P=0.021$) showed that patients lost weight when they received lamotrigine relative to the weight gained when they received gabapentin. In contrast to the weight gain observed during treatment with gabapentin, patients lost weight while receiving lamotrigine therapy during this 6-week trial. This relatively weight-neutral profile is a potential advantage for lamotrigine over other mood stabilizers, such as lithium or divalproex.

This study suggests that lamotrigine monotherapy is superior to both gabapentin and placebo in patients with refractory mood disorders. Although crossover designs have the potential for producing carryover and other confounding effects, this did not appear to occur in this analysis and did not affect the interpretation of the outcome data based on a variety of considerations. These data suggest that the response rates were not confounded by the treatment phase, nor were they influenced by carryover effects on the severity of illness. Nonetheless, the 6-week treatment phases and total study period of 18 weeks is a short period to assess the efficacy or persistence of response. A very high percentage (92%) of the bipolar patients in this sample had rapid cycling, which is substantially greater than the general population estimates of this course specifier (DSM-IV-TR). Both refractory unipolar and bipolar patients were included in this preliminary study. In addition, the direct application of these preliminary monotherapy results to community treatment guidelines is limited, given that a combination treatment is the norm and monotherapy regimens are rarely used in clinical practice.

In the first multicenter, double-blind, placebo-controlled study of lamotrigine in rapid-cycling bipolar disorder, 182 of 324 (56%) patients with rapid cycling responded to treatment with open label lamotrigine and were then randomized to the double-blind, randomized phase of the study (Calabrese et al. 2000). Open label treatment was initiated in 324 patients meeting DSM-IV criteria for rapid-cycling bipolar disorder, with 182 stabilized patients later randomly assigned to the double-blind maintenance phase. For patients entering the open stabilization phase, the mean age was 38 years with a female:male ratio of 3:2. The percentage of bipolar I subtype was 69%. At study entry, 57% of patients were in a depressed phase, 20% were hypomanic or manic, 18% were euthymic, and 5% had mixed states. The mean number of mood episodes in the 12 months before study entry was 6.3. The lifetime prevalence of psychosis was 27%, and percentage of patients with prior suicide attempts was 36%. The majority of enrolled subjects had been previously exposed to lithium, divalproex, and antidepressants. About one-quarter of the patients had taken carbamazepine or antipsychotics in the past, but less than 1% had prior exposure to lamotrigine. Concomitant psychiatric medications at study entry included lithium (19%), carbamazepine (4%), divalproex (19%), antidepressants (30%), and antipsychotics (7%). Although the most commonly prescribed lifetime medications at the time of study entry were antidepressants, only 36% of patients reported positive response to these agents.

During the open-label treatment phase, lamotrigine was added to the current psychotropic regimen and titrated to clinical effect. Stabilized patients were tapered off treatment with other psychotropics and randomly assigned to lamotrigine or placebo monotherapy (in a 1:1 ratio) for 6 months after being stratified for bipolar I or II disorder. Lamotrigine dosage was titrated in the 6-week preliminary phase to a target dosage of 200 mg/day. After week 5, lamotrigine dosage increases were allowed in increments of 100 mg/week up to a maximum dosage of 300 mg/day. In the randomized phase, the double-blind medication dosage was also flexible and varied from 100 mg/day to 500 mg/day. The average daily lamotrigine dosage was 288±94 mg.

The primary outcome measure was time to additional pharmacotherapy for emerging symptoms of any mood episode. Secondary outcome measures included survival in the study, percentage of patients stable without relapse for 6 months, and changes in scores on the Global Assessment Scale (GAS) and the Clinical Global Impression–Severity of Illness Scale (CGI-S). Kaplan-Meier methodology was used to analyze survival data, and median times to survival were calculated. Survival analyses were performed for each bipolar subtype. The percentage of patients stable without relapse for 6 months was analyzed using the Cochran-Mantel-Haenszel chi-square test. Clinical efficacy scales (CGI-S, GAS) were evaluated using analysis of variance (ANOVA) at an $\alpha=0.05$ level of significance using both observed and last-observation-carried-forward (LOCF) data.

Treatment groups during the randomized phase ($N=182$) were similar with respect to age, sex, race, medical history, psychiatric history, prior treatments, response to treatments, and current psychiatric state. The majority of patients were classified as having bipolar I disorder (71%). A comparison of bipolar I and II patients showed no difference on multiple key parameters. However, compared with bipolar II patients, bipolar I patients had a greater prevalence of suicide attempts (40% versus 28%) and average number of lifetime hospitalizations (2.3 versus 0.7). Forty-nine placebo-arm patients (56%) and 45 lamotrigine-arm patients (50%) required additional pharmacotherapy for emerging symptoms of a mood episode. The difference between the two treatment groups in time to additional pharmacotherapy did not achieve statistical significance.

The median survival times to intervention were 18 weeks for lamotrigine and 12 weeks for placebo. When survival in study (any premature discontinuation, including for additional pharmacotherapy) was evaluated, the difference between the treatment groups was significant ($P=0.04$). For survival in study, the median survival times were 14 weeks for lamotrigine and 8 weeks for placebo. Time to additional pharmacotherapy and survival in study did not yield significant differences between lamotrigine and placebo in patients with bipolar I disorder. When time to additional pharmacotherapy was evaluated, a trend toward significance ($P=0.07$) was found in the separation between placebo and lamotrigine. Median survival time without additional pharmacotherapy for the bipolar II subtype was 17 weeks for lamotrigine and 7 weeks for placebo. The overall survival in study analysis yielded a significant separation between treatment groups ($P=0.01$). Median overall survival was 15 weeks for lamotrigine and 4 weeks for placebo. The majority of those patients (80%) requiring additional pharmacotherapy were treated for depressive symptoms; 20% were treated for emerging manic, hypomanic, or mixed symptoms.

The percentage of patients who completed the 6-month randomized phase clinically stable on monotherapy without evidence of relapse into hypomania, mania, or depression was significantly greater in the lamotrigine group than in the placebo group. Of the 60 patients who were stable for 6 months of monotherapy, 37 of 90 (41%) were in the lamotrigine group compared with 23 of 87 (26%) in the placebo group ($P=0.03$). The difference between lamotrigine versus placebo was not statistically significant for the bipolar I subtype but was significant (46% vs. 18%, respectively; $P=0.04$) for the bipolar II subtype. The CGI-S and GAS were used to provide additional measures of clinical stability. For the overall study population and the bipolar I subtype, there was no statistically significant difference between treatment groups in CGI-S change from baseline scores using LOCF. For the bipolar II subtype, trends toward statistically significant differences ($P<0.10$) favoring the lamotrigine group were observed in CGI-S scores compared with the placebo group at weeks 6 and 12. No statistically significant differences favoring lamotrigine were observed between groups in GAS change from baseline scores in the general cohort of patients (LOCF). Significant differences favoring lamotrigine were noted at weeks 3, 6, and 12 in the bipolar II subtype; however, no significant differences were noted at any time for the bipolar I subtype. There were no significant differences observed in the change from baseline LOCF analyses at any point for the 17-item Hamilton Rating Scale for Depression (Ham-D) or the YMRS.

The most common adverse events ($\geq$10%) observed during the open stabilization phase were headache, infection, influenza, nausea, dream abnormality, dizziness, and rash. In the randomized phase, 122 patients (67% lamotrigine; 68% placebo) experienced adverse events, and the most common adverse events were headache, nausea, infection, pain, and accidental injury. Lamotrigine-related rash occurred in 8% of patients during open stabilization and in no patients in the randomized phase. There were no serious rashes during either phase of the study, and no patients required hospitalization for a rash. Lamotrigine-treated patients did not appear to gain any significant weight as a group.

The small sample size limits the generalizability of this study's conclusions, because the actual enrollment of fewer than 100 patients per treatment arm limited the power of the primary outcome analysis to approximately 0.47. In contrast, the analysis of survival in study was retrospectively determined to have been powered at approximately 0.83. The design of this study did not permit an analysis of time to relapse into a full episode of depression, hypomania, or mania since patients were withdrawn at the first signs of relapse. In addition, this study enrolled a higher proportion of patients with bipolar I disorder than is thought to occur in the rapid-cycling population. Lamotrigine was well tolerated in this study and the type and frequency of adverse events were comparable to placebo.

In this study, lamotrigine demonstrated efficacy in the prevention of the recurrence of mood symptoms over a 6-month period in recently stabilized rapid-cycling bipolar patients. The results of this study suggest that lamotrigine may be a well-tolerated and effective mood stabilizer with prophylactic properties when used as monotherapy in some patients with rapid-cycling bipolar disorder. Lamotrigine may be an especially effective mood stabilizer for patients diagnosed with bipolar II disorder.

Practical Considerations

The risk of Stevens-Johnson syndrome or toxic epidermal necrolysis associated with lamotrigine use is recognized as an issue that certainly deserves continued awareness and caution. However, most of the published cases of severe rashes during lamotrigine therapy occurred before current recommendations for a slow initial taper were introduced. Benign rash has occurred in 9% (108/1,198) of patients randomized to lamotrigine versus 8% (80/1,056) of patients randomized to placebo in pivotal multicenter, double-blind, placebo-controlled bipolar trials. In all mood disorder trials conducted to date, the rate of serious rash (defined as requiring both drug discontinuation and hospitalization) has been 0.06% (2/3,153) on lamotrigine and 0.09% (1/1,053) on placebo (Calabrese et al. 2001c). Stevens-Johnson syndrome or toxic epidermal necrolysis were not observed in any patient given lamotrigine in these trials.

A low starting dosage and gradual titration of lamotrigine minimize the risk of serious rash. When prescribed in the absence of enzyme inhibitors (divalproex) or inducers (carbamazepine), the recommended dosing is 25 mg/day for weeks 1 and 2, 50 mg/day for weeks 3 and 4, 100 mg/day for week 5, and then 200 mg/day thereafter. Lamotrigine dosing should be doubled in the presence of carbamazepine and halved when the drug is co-administered with divalproex.

Olanzapine

Evidence

In the first randomized, parallel-group, placebo-controlled trial to evaluate the efficacy of olanzapine in bipolar I depression, the efficacy of olanzapine was evaluated in patients with and without rapid cycling. The sample size of the rapid-cycling subgroup included 132 patients assigned to placebo, 142 to olanzapine monotherapy, and 34 to the combination of fluoxetine plus olanzapine. Overall, significant improvement in Montgomery-Åsberg Depression Rating Scale (MADRS) total scores compared with placebo at final assessment occurred in the olanzapine monotherapy group and the group combining fluoxetine plus olanzapine. However, the combination therapy arm was superior to both olanzapine monotherapy and placebo, with significant improvement occurring as early as the first week of treatment. Whereas the magnitude of the overall clinical effect size was small for olanzapine monotherapy (0.32), the effect size for the olanzapine-fluoxetine combination was moderately large (0.68). In patients with rapid cycling, the combination of olanzapine and fluoxetine resulted in a statistically significant decrease ($P<0.05$) in MADRS total score at week 8 compared with the olanzapine monotherapy and placebo-treated groups, suggesting better antidepressant effect for the olanzapine-fluoxetine combination (mean change in MADRS scores: –15.6 for the combination group compared with only –10.5 and –10.3 in the olanzapine monotherapy and placebo groups, respectively). In patients without rapid cycling, both the olanzapine-fluoxetine combination and olanzapine monotherapy groups had significant decreases in total MADRS score (–18.1 and –14.0) compared to placebo (–8.7). The difference between decreases seen in MADRS scores in the combination and monotherapy groups was statistically significant ($P<0.05$), suggesting that although olanzapine has antidepressant effects in non–rapid cyclers compared with placebo, the combination of olanzapine-fluoxetine has higher antidepressant efficacy in this population. Active treatment, either as monotherapy or in combination with fluoxetine, was not associated with an elevated level of treatment-emergent mania compared with placebo (Tohen et al. 2003).

Placebo-controlled, randomized, double-blind trials of olanzapine in acute bipolar mania have proven efficacy for olanzapine over placebo in patients exhibiting a broad spectrum of bipolar variables, including recent rapid cycling (Baldessarini et al. 2003). Olanzapine was shown to be effective in reducing symptoms of mania in patients with bipolar disorder with a history of a rapid-cycling course (Sanger et al. 2003). Pooled data from these two (Baldessarini et al. 2003; Sanger et al. 2003) placebo-controlled, randomized, double-blind trials of olanzapine in mania plus open 12-month follow-up extension have also been recently analyzed, specifically looking at clinical and outcome measures in rapid-cycling patients (n=90) compared with non–rapid-cycling patients (n=164). Rapid-cycling bipolar patients were significantly more likely to be younger; to have a greater number of previous episodes and hospitalizations; and to have less severe manic symptoms, more severe depressive symptoms, and less psychotic symptoms. They were also more likely to have a history of substance abuse; a family history of bipolar disorder, depression, and substance abuse; and offspring depression. By intention-to-treat measure, they were more likely to respond short-term to either olanzapine or placebo than non–rapid-cycling patients, but in the long term they were more likely to relapse. Olanzapine, however, improved the overall outcome of both rapid-cycling and non–rapid-cycling patients. These authors concluded that rapid-cycling patients show substantial clinical differences compared with non–rapid-cycling patients. They are also more likely to be short-term responders when enrolled in a clinical trial, thus increasing placebo response, although their long-term outcome is worse (Vieta et al. 2004).

Practical Considerations

As of early 2005, olanzapine was the only atypical antipsychotic with approval from the U.S Food and Drug Administration for long-term management of bipolar disorder. As with the common clinical practice of continuing antipsychotics given alone or in conjunction with mood stabilizers for acute mania beyond the remission of the acute episode, the need to continue olanzapine must be reassessed given the concerns of potential weight gain and metabolic and endocrine dysfunction seen with atypical antipsychotics. In addition, therapy with olanzapine is sometimes complicated by other common side effects such as dizziness, constipation, increased liver enzyme, akathisia, and postural hypotension.

During acute manic episodes associated with rapid-cycling bipolar disorder, experience suggests that if olanzapine monotherapy is attempted, a minimum dosage of 15–20 mg/day is required. Adjunctive or combined use of olanzapine with another antimanic agent, such as lithium or divalproex, may involve somewhat lower olanzapine dosages. Management of acute depressive episodes with olanzapine or olanzapine-fluoxetine combination may require 5–20 mg/day of olanzapine. Long-term prophylactic dosing for rapid-cycling bipolar disorder can be variable; patients with severe or intractable type I rapid-cycling bipolar disorder may benefit more from a sustained higher dosage of olanzapine, whereas those with less severe manic presentations or type II disorder may remain on lower dosages, increasing olanzapine only when hypomanic/manic symptoms begin to emerge in a form of antimanic "rescue" therapy.

The implication for treatment of rapid-cycling bipolar disorder with olanzapine draws a parallel to the profile of lamotrigine as a putative antidepressant for depressive phases, with olanzapine offering superior control of more severe manic phases than lamotrigine and potentially protecting against mood acceleration or cycling if traditional antidepressants must be co-administered. Combination with antidepressants, such as fluoxetine, may be necessary in depressed and fragile patients, although data to support this practice are limited among rapid-cycling cohorts. Combining olanzapine with other mood stabilizers, such as lithium or divalproex, may enhance the efficacy of these treatment strategies in all phases of bipolar disorder. However, additive side effects such as sedation and weight gain may substantially limit practical use of this combination therapy beyond short-term control of accelerations in rapid cycling.

Quetiapine

Evidence

In the first randomized, parallel-group, placebo-controlled trial to evaluate the efficacy of quetiapine in bipolar I and II depression, the efficacy of quetiapine was evaluated in patients with and without rapid-cycling bipolar disorder. The sample size of the rapid-cycling subgroup included 35 patients assigned to placebo, 31 to quetiapine 600 mg/day, and 42 to quetiapine 300 mg/day. Overall, significant improvement in MADRS total scores compared with placebo at final assessment occurred with quetiapine treatment regardless of the presence of rapid cycling. In patients with rapid cycling at week 8, quetiapine 300 mg/day and 600 mg/day treatment both led to a mean decrease in MADRS total score that was significantly different from placebo (mean change in MADRS scores: quetiapine 300 mg/day=−18.6, quetiapine 600 mg/day=−17.7, placebo=−9.9; $P<0.01$ for both treatment groups compared with placebo). In patients without rapid cycling, the mean decrease in MADRS total score at week 8 was also significantly greater in both quetiapine treatment groups compared with placebo (Calabrese et al. 2004). These findings suggest that quetiapine at dosages of 300–600 mg/day may be effective in treating acute bipolar I or II depression, and equally effective in rapid-cycling and non–rapid-cycling patients.

As noted in Chapter 2, unfortunately, patients with rapid cycling were excluded from the pivotal double-blind, placebo-controlled quetiapine monotherapy and adjunctive therapy acute mania studies, limiting our ability to appreciate the utility of quetiapine for acute manic symptoms in patients with rapid cycling.

There are additional reports that may suggest efficacy for quetiapine in rapid-cycling patients, either as monotherapy or as add-on therapy. An open-label prospective study of 40 patients with type I rapid-cycling bipolar disorder on quetiapine treatment (mean dosage 159.4 ± 161.5 mg/day), with or without adjunctive mood stabilizer, suggested that this atypical antipsychotic is effective as add-on and monotherapy and is well tolerated (Ghaemi et al. 2001).

Interim analysis included 16 subjects entered into the study with any mood symptomatology severe enough to require added medication intervention. Eight subjects were on concomitant lithium and/or divalproex or concomitant lamotrigine. Only one patient was taking an antidepressant (fluoxetine). Preliminary data analysis at weeks 4, 8, and 12 indicated improvement in both Ham-D and YMRS scores. At week 8, depressive symptom improvement trended towards statistical significance, but not at week 12. Manic symptom improvement was statistically significant at weeks 4 and 12. CGI-BP ratings indicated improvement in both manic and depressive symptoms for week 2 onwards, with statistical significance for manic symptoms at week 4, and overall bipolar illness at weeks 4 and 8. Weight change was minimal, with a mean of 1.2 lbs lost at 15 weeks of follow-up. Preliminary conclusions suggested that at 3-month follow-up quetiapine improves rapid-cycling symptoms in bipolar disorder.

A second report supported these findings, suggesting quetiapine has efficacy as an add-on therapy to other mood stabilizers for rapid-cycling bipolar disorder (Vieta et al. 2002). The required dosages of quetiapine may differ substantially for acute phase of illness: 720 ± 84 mg/day for mania versus 183 ± 29 mg/day for depression. This report also suggested quetiapine has preferential efficacy for manic episodes over depressive ones, although unpublished data have shown robust antidepressant response to quetiapine (300–600 mg/day) in non–rapid-cycling bipolar I depression (Calabrese et al., in press).

Practical Considerations

The relatively decreased frequency and severity of weight gain with quetiapine compared with olanzapine makes it an attractive alternative among atypical antipsychotics and other agents for the management of rapid-cycling bipolar disorder. The most common side effects are somnolence, dizziness, dry mouth, postural hypotension, and elevated alanine aminotransferase (serum glutamate pyruvate transaminase) levels.

Management of acute mania with quetiapine in rapid-cycling bipolar disorder can be accomplished using the recommended labeling guidelines of titration in 100 mg/day increments from 100 mg/day in divided dosing on day 1 to 400 mg/day on day 4. Further incremental increases of 200 mg/day up to 800 mg/day may be needed in some patients, with an average therapeutic dosage in most patients being 600 mg/day. Dosages of 300–600 mg/day have been reported to be effective during acutely depressed phases of bipolar I disorder in patients with and without rapid cycling.

Conclusions

Most of the literature supports the impression that a recent history of rapid-cycling bipolar disorder is a general predictor of poor long-term outcome, essentially functioning as a nonspecific indicator of severity. This conclusion is in some contrast to prior impressions that rapid cycling was a specific predictor of poor outcome to some (lithium), but not other (divalproex) pharmacotherapies. Highly recurrent treatment-refractory depression appears to be the hallmark of rapid-cycling bipolar disorder, and the majority of patients appear to be either not diagnosed or incorrectly treated for recurrent major depression. There are no controlled data that support the use of the conventional antidepressants in the short- or long-term treatment of patients with rapid cycling. Lithium, lamotrigine, fluoxetine-olanzapine combination, and quetiapine have been shown to have acute efficacy in the treatment of patients with rapid cycling based on controlled trials. The addition of lamotrigine to our long-term pharmacotherapeutic armamentarium appears to be a helpful adjunct, particularly when used with an agent that stabilizes "mood from above baseline," and it is particularly well suited for treatment-refractory depressive mood states. In the short-term, patients with rapid cycling enrolled in acute clinical trials are more likely to experience short-term response, thus increasing placebo response, although their long-term outcome is worse.

References

Akiskal HS, Bourgeois ML, Angst J, et al: Re-evaluating the prevalence of and diagnostic composition within the broad clinical spectrum of bipolar disorders. J Affect Disord 59 (suppl 1):S5–S30, 2000

American Psychiatric Association: Diagnostic and Statistical Manual of Mental Disorders, 4th Edition. Washington, DC, American Psychiatric Association, 1994

American Psychiatric Association: Diagnostic and Statistical Manual of Mental Disorders, 4th Edition, Text Revision. Washington, DC, American Psychiatric Association, 2000

Angst J, Sellaro R: Historical perspectives and natural history of bipolar disorder. Biol Psychiatry 48:445–457, 2000

Baldessarini RJ, Tondo L, Floris G, et al: Effects of rapid cycling on response to lithium maintenance treatment in 360 bipolar I and II disorder patients. J Affect Disord 61:13–22, 2000

Baldessarini RJ, Tondo L, Hennen J, et al: Is lithium still worth using? An update of selected recent research. Harv Rev Psychiatry 10:59–75, 2002

Baldessarini RJ, Hennen J, Wilson M, et al: Olanzapine versus placebo in acute mania: treatment responses in subgroups. J Clin Psychopharmacol 23:370–376, 2003

Bauer MS, Calabrese JR, Dunner DL, et al: Multisite data reanalysis of the validity of rapid cycling as a course modifier for bipolar disorder in DSM-IV. Am J Psychiatry 151:506–515, 1994

Bowden CL: Clinical correlates of therapeutic response in bipolar disorder. J Affect Disord 67:257–265, 2001

Bowden CL, Calabrese JR, McElroy SL, et al: The efficacy of lamotrigine in rapid cycling and non-rapid cycling patients with bipolar disorder. Biol Psychiatry 45:953–958, 1999

Calabrese JR, Delucchi GA: Spectrum of efficacy of valproate in 55 patients with rapid-cycling bipolar disorder. Am J Psychiatry 147:431–434, 1990

Calabrese JR, Markovitz PJ, Kimmel SE, et al: Spectrum of efficacy of valproate in 78 rapid-cycling bipolar patients. J Clin Psychopharmacol 12:53S–56S, 1992

Calabrese JR, Bowden CL, Woyshville M: Lithium and anticonvulsants in the treatment of bipolar disorder, in Psychopharmacology: The Third Generation of Progress. Editd by Meltzer HY. New York, Raven, 1994, pp 1019–1111

Calabrese JR, Bowden CL, Sachs GS, et al: A double-blind placebo-controlled study of lamotrigine monotherapy in outpatients with bipolar I depression: Lamictal 602 Study Group. J Clin Psychiatry 60:79–88, 1999

Calabrese JR, Suppes T, Bowden CL, et al: A double-blind, placebo-controlled, prophylaxis study of lamotrigine in rapid-cycling bipolar disorder: Lamictal 614 Study Group. J Clin Psychiatry 61:841–850, 2000

Calabrese JR, Shelton MD, Bowden CL, et al: Bipolar rapid cycling: focus on depression as its hallmark. J Clin Psychiatry 62 (suppl 14):34–41, 2001a

Calabrese JR, Shelton MD, Rapport DJ, et al: Current research on rapid cycling bipolar disorder and its treatment. J Affect Disord 67:241–255, 2001b

Calabrese JR, Suppes T, Swann AC, et al: Lamotrigine and rash: a review of evidence from double-blind, placebo-controlled trials in bipolar disorder patients. Presented at the annual meeting of the American College of Neuropsychopharmacology, Waikoloa, HI, December 2001c

Calabrese JR, McFadden W, McCoy R, et al: Double-blind, placebo-controlled study of quetiapine in bipolar depression. Presented at the 157th annual meeting of the American Psychiatric Association, New York, May 2004

Calabrese JR, Keck PE, MacFadden W, et al: A randomized, double-blind, placebo-controlled trial of quetiapine in the treatment of bipolar I or II depression. Am J Psychiatry, in press

Calabrese JR, Shelton MD, Rapport DJ, et al: A 20-month, double-blind, maintenance trial of lithium versus divalproex in rapid-cycling bipolar disorder. Am J Psychiatry, in press

Denicoff KD, Smith-Jackson EE, Disney ER, et al: Comparative prophylactic efficacy of lithium, carbamazepine, and the combination in bipolar disorder. J Clin Psychiatry 58:470–478, 1997

Di Costanzo E, Schifano F: Lithium alone or in combination with carbamazepine for the treatment of rapid-cycling bipolar affective disorder. Acta Psychiatr Scand 83:456–459, 1991

Dunner DL, Fieve RR: Clinical factors in lithium carbonate prophylaxis failure. Arch Gen Psychiatry 30:229–233, 1974

Frye MA, Ketter TA, Kimbrell TA, et al: A placebo-controlled study of lamotrigine and gabapentin monotherapy in refractory mood disorders. J Clin Psychopharmacol 20:607–614, 2000

Ghaemi SN, Goldberg JF, Ko J, et al: Seroquel treatment of rapid cycling bipolar disorder: an open prospective study. Presented at the Fourth International Conference on Bipolar Disorder, Pittsburgh, PA, June 2001

Goodwin FK: Rationale for long-term treatment of bipolar disorder and evidence for long-term lithium treatment. J Clin Psychiatry 63 (suppl 10):5–12, 2002

Joffe RT: Carbamazepine, lithium, and life course of bipolar affective disorder. Am J Psychiatry 148:1270–1271, 1991

Kleindienst N, Greil W: Inter-episodic morbidity and drop-out under carbamazepine and lithium in the maintenance treatment of bipolar disorder. Psychol Med 32:493–501, 2002

Kraepelin E: Psychiatrie III, Klinische Psychiatrie II. Leipzig, Germany, Verlag von Johann Ambrosius Barth, 1913

Kukopulos A, Reginaldi D, Laddomada P, et al: Course of the manic-depressive cycle and changes caused by treatment. Pharmakopsychiatr Neuropsychopharmakol 13:156–167, 1980

Maj M, Starace F, Nolfe G, et al: Minimum plasma lithium levels required for effective prophylaxis in DSM III bipolar disorder: a prospective study. Pharmacopsychiatry 19:420–423, 1986

Maj M, Magliano L, Pirozzi R, et al: Validity of rapid cycling as a course specifier for bipolar disorder. Am J Psychiatry 151:1015–1019, 1994

Maj M, Pirozzi R, Magliano L, et al: Long-term outcome of lithium prophylaxis in bipolar disorder: a 5-year prospective study of 402 patients at a lithium clinic. Am J Psychiatry 155:30–35, 1998

Maj M, Pirozzi R, Formicola AM, et al: Reliability and validity of four alternative definitions of rapid-cycling bipolar disorder. Am J Psychiatry 156:1421–1424, 1999

Okuma T: Effects of carbamazepine and lithium on affective disorders. Neuropsychobiology 27:138–145, 1993

Post RM, Uhde TW, Roy-Byrne PP, et al: Correlates of antimanic response to carbamazepine. Psychiatry Res 21:71–83, 1987

Post RM, Frye MA, Denicoff KD, et al: Emerging trends in the treatment of rapid cycling bipolar disorder: a selected review. Bipolar Disord 2:305–315, 2000

Sanger TM, Tohen M, Vieta E, et al: Olanzapine in the acute treatment of bipolar I disorder with a history of rapid cycling. J Affect Disord 73:155–161, 2003

Sharma V, Persad E, Mazmanian D, et al: Treatment of rapid cycling bipolar disorder with combination therapy of valproate and lithium. Can J Psychiatry 38:137–139, 1993

Swann AC: Prediction of treatment response in acute mania: controlled clinical trials with divalproex. Encephale 27:277–279, 2001

Swann AC, Bowden CL, Calabrese JR, et al: Mania: differential effects of previous depressive and manic episodes on response to treatment. Acta Psychiatr Scand 101:444–451, 2000

Tohen M, Vieta E, Calabrese JR, et al: Efficacy of olanzapine and olanzapine-fluoxetine combination in the treatment of bipolar I depression. Arch Gen Psychiatry 60:1079–1088, 2003

Tondo L, Baldessarini RJ, Hennen J, et al: Lithium maintenance treatment of depression and mania in bipolar I and bipolar II disorders. Am J Psychiatry 155:638–645, 1998

Tondo L, Baldessarini RJ, Floris G: Long-term clinical effectiveness of lithium maintenance treatment in types I and II bipolar disorders. Br J Psychiatry 178(suppl):184–190, 2001

Tondo L, Hennen J, Baldessarini RJ: Rapid-cycling bipolar disorder: effects of long-term treatments. Acta Psychiatr Scand 108:4–14, 2003

Tremont G, Stern RA: Use of thyroid hormone to diminish the cognitive side effects of psychiatric treatment. Psychopharmacol Bull 33:273–280, 1997

Vieta E, Parramon G, Padrell E, et al: Quetiapine in the treatment of rapid cycling bipolar disorder. Bipolar Disord 4:335–340, 2002

Vieta E, Calabrese JR, Tohen M, et al: Comparison of rapid-cycling and non-rapid-cycling bipolar I manic patients during treatment with olanzapine: analysis of pooled data. J Clin Psychiatry 65:1420–1428, 2004

Viguera AC, Baldessarini RJ, Tondo L: Response to lithium maintenance treatment in bipolar disorders: comparison of women and men. Bipolar Disord 3:245–252, 2001

Walden J, Schaerer L, Schloesser S, et al: An open longitudinal study of patients with bipolar rapid cycling treated with lithium or lamotrigine for mood stabilization. Bipolar Disord 2:336–339, 2000

Wehr TA, Sack DA, Rosenthal NE, et al: Rapid cycling affective disorder: contributing factors and treatment responses in 51 patients. Am J Psychiatry 145:179–184, 1988

Chapter 6

Treatment of Children and Adolescents With Bipolar Disorder

Kiki D. Chang, M.D.
Meghan Howe, M.S.W.
Diana I. Simeonova, Dipl.-Psych.

Although the past decade has seen impressive advances in the identification of children and adolescents with bipolar disorder, it remains imperative that even more progress be made in developing evidenced-based treatments, indications, and guidelines for treating these youth. It is becoming clear that youth with bipolar disorder require an integrated treatment program involving medications, psychotherapy, and educational interventions. However, the exact nature and best way to implement and coordinate these interventions remain to be determined. Specifically, there is no medication with U.S. Food and Drug Administration (FDA) approval for the treatment of bipolar disorder in children and adolescents. Nevertheless, existing data support the use of specific medications in this population. This chapter discusses the current treatment modalities used in pediatric bipolar disorder that are supported by empirical data. We primarily focus on pharmacotherapy, because there is more information in this area than for other interventions, but we also include emerging data regarding promising psychotherapeutic interventions for this population. Although it is premature to include specific recommendations for educational interventions, it is crucial that clinicians not overlook the educational needs of these children. We conclude with a discussion of early intervention and prevention of bipolar disorder in youth, an area in very early stages of development with the potential to attenuate or perhaps even avoid the burden of fully developed bipolar disorder in children, adolescents, and even adults.

Pharmacotherapy

In contrast to adult bipolar disorder (American Psychiatric Association 2002; Keck et al. 2004), current treatment guidelines for pediatric bipolar disorder are only beginning to emerg. However, published reviews have summarized optimal treatment approaches for this population (Chang and Ketter 2001; Davanzo and McCracken 2000; Kowatch and DelBello 2003). Medication interventions, as for adults, are essential, but optimal pharmacological treatment algorithms based on empirical data remain to be established. Therefore, this chapter reviews the sort of current empirical evidence for the efficacy of different psychotropic medications in pediatric bipolar disorder that clinicians need in order to provide evidence-based management.

In the absence of adequate placebo-controlled studies, treatment approaches for the pediatric population have been largely derived from those for adults that are described elsewhere in this volume. This is far from ideal, because children possess family, psychosocial, and neurobiological environments far distinct from those of adults. Fortunately, controlled studies are increasingly being conducted in pediatric bipolar disorder and will undoubtedly bring additional empirical data to guide treatment. Data regarding children are largely concerned with treatment of acute mania. Treatment for acute bipolar depression and maintenance treatment are being increasingly studied in adults, as described in Chapters 3 and 4, respectively, but such data in children are still lacking. For example, it is unclear exactly how long to continue treatment with mood stabilizers in children with bipolar disorder. One study of adolescents with bipolar disorder reported an 18-month relapse rate of 92% with lithium discontinuation compared with 37% with continued lithium treatment (Strober et al. 1990). Therefore, it appears prudent to continue mood stabilizer treatment for at least the first 18 months after an initial manic episode. However, based on the chronic and relapsing nature of pediatric bipolar disorder (Geller et al. 2002), most children with bipolar disorder will likely require even longer-term treatment. Further studies of long-term mood stabilizer treatment and optimal management of bipolar depression in children and adolescents are needed to help inform clinicians.

Lithium and Anticonvulsants

Lithium

Lithium is one of the more extensively studied medications for pediatric mania. Multiple open trials suggest that lithium may be efficacious in pediatric mania (DeLong 1978; Hassanyeh and Davison 1980; Hsu 1986; Kafantaris et al. 2003; Kowatch et al. 2000; McKnew et al. 1981; Strober et al. 1988; Varanka et al. 1988; Wagner et al. 2002). The first published double-blind, placebo-controlled study of a mood stabilizer in pediatric bipolar disorder reported on the treatment of 25 adolescents with bipolar disorder or major depressive disorder and strong family histories of bipolar disorder (Geller et al. 1998). Subjects were treated either with lithium (mean dosage $1,733 \pm 428$ mg/day, mean plasma concentration 0.88 ± 0.27 mEq/L) or placebo over a 6-week period. Six of 13 participants in the lithium group had a significant decrease in manic symptoms as judged by Children's Global Assessment Scale scores compared with only 1 of 12 in the placebo group ($P=0.046$). In addition, substance abuse decreased significantly in the adolescents taking lithium compared with those given placebo. Patients given lithium experienced significantly greater thirst, polyuria, nausea, vomiting, diarrhea, and dizziness than those taking placebo.

Empirical evidence for the use of lithium for maintenance treatment of bipolar disorder in children and adolescents is limited. There is only one longer-term study of adolescents with pediatric bipolar disorder, which found that 92% of the participants openly discontinuing lithium had a manic relapse within 18 months compared with 38% of those who continued taking lithium (Strober et al. 1990). Furthermore, despite its history of efficacy as a first-line mood stabilizer, lithium may be ineffective in some pediatric populations. Adolescents with bipolar disorder and a prepubertal onset of any psychiatric disorder (Strober et al. 1988), specifically attention-deficit/hyperactivity disorder (ADHD; Strober et al. 1998), may be less likely to respond to lithium. Other possible indicators of lithium nonresponse in pediatric bipolar disorder include presence of a comorbid personality disorder (Kutcher et al. 1990) and mixed states (Himmelhoch and Garfinkel 1986). The latter may be a particularly significant limitation, because these states are commonly observed in pediatric bipolar disorder (Findling et al. 2001; Geller et al. 1995).

Valproate

Although there have been no published placebo-controlled studies of the use of valproate in pediatric bipolar disorder, open-label trials suggest possible efficacy in pediatric populations (Kowatch et al. 2000; Papatheodorou and Kutcher 1993; Papatheodorou et al. 1995; Wagner et al. 2002; West et al. 1994). Interestingly, overall response rates from these studies resemble those for lithium (66% for lithium and 65% for valproate). In a recent open study, valproate monotherapy (mean dosage 813 ± 338 mg/day, mean plasma concentration 83.4 ± 25.4 µg/mL) yielded symptomatic improvement in 22 of 40 (55%) children and adolescents (ages 7–19 years) with bipolar mania as measured by at least a 50% decrease in Mania Rating Scale scores (Wagner et al. 2002). Adverse effects reported during the 2- to 8-week trial included nausea, vomiting, headache, and somnolence. Controlled maintenance treatment data with valproate in children and adolescents are lacking; however, a retrospective chart review of 15 children and adolescents with bipolar disorder (mean age 13 years) treated with open long-term divalproex (mean 1.4 years) indicated moderate to marked global improvement in 8 patients (53%) (Henry et al. 2003). The mean dosage was 966 mg/day and mean plasma concentration was 79.4 ± 23.1 µg/mL, with the most common adverse effect being weight gain.

Early data indicated that divalproex might be more effective than lithium for treating mixed mania or rapid-cycling states in adults (Calabrese et al. 1993), but, as noted in Chapter 5, later reports have been less encouraging regarding efficacy in rapid cycling, and it is not clear whether this equivocal finding applies in pediatric bipolar disorder. A historical case control comparison indicated a greater risk of relapse for adolescents with mixed mania on lithium compared with divalproex (Davanzo and McCracken 2000). It is also unclear if younger children with bipolar disorder respond to valproate treatment. However, one case series described good response to divalproex (250–500 mg/day) in nine young children (ages 2–7) with symptoms suggestive of mania (Mota-Castillo et al. 2001).

Carbamazepine

Although a proprietary extended-release formulation of carbamazepine was recently approved for the treatment of acute mania in adults, the use of carbamazepine in pediatric bipolar disorder has not been studied extensively. However, limited empirical evidence from studies of patients with mixed diagnoses and case reports support its use as a mood stabilizer. Effective treatment of adolescents with bipolar disorder has been reported in cases of carbamazepine monotherapy (Woolston 1999) as well as in adjunctive therapy with lithium (Hsu 1986). Open carbamazepine monotherapy (mean serum concentration 7.1 ± 1.8 µg/mL) helped 4 of 13 children and adolescents with mania (Kowatch et al. 2000). The majority of side effects were mild to moderate, with the most common being nausea. Because of concerns about the risk for serious adverse effects such as aplastic anemia and the paucity of studies in childhood mania, carbamazepine is not a first-line medication for pediatric bipolar disorder. However, given the extensive data suggesting safety in pediatric epilepsy and efficacy in adults with bipolar disorder, studies of carbamazepine in pediatric bipolar disorder are warranted.

Gabapentin

Evidence for the efficacy of gabapentin in the treatment of pediatric bipolar disorder is meager and uncontrolled. In case reports, open gabapentin (200–1,500 mg/day) helped an adolescent (Soutullo et al. 1998) and a child with bipolar disorder (Hamrin and Bailey 2001). Despite its good tolerability (Khurana et al. 1996; McLean

1995), adverse behavioral effects have been noted in children, including irritability and worsening of aggressive behavior (Lee et al. 1996), and have been included in the product information.

Lamotrigine

As of early 2005, there were no published placebo-controlled studies of lamotrigine in children or adolescents with bipolar disorder. Seven adolescents with rapid cycling or refractory bipolar depression participated in a 6-week open-label study of adjunctive lamotrigine treatment that included adult subjects (Kusumakar and Yatham 1997). By week 4, 72% of the subjects responded and by week 6, 63% were considered remitted. In this study, the main adverse effects were tremor and headache. Despite a more rapid than recommended titration and adjunctive treatment with valproate in some participants, there were no rashes. A higher incidence of serious rash in children compared with adults taking lamotrigine has been reported in the past (Dooley et al. 1996; Messenheimer et al. 2000). As in adults, increased risk of rash was considered related to higher initial dosing and more rapid titration than currently recommended, and lack of adjustment of dosage for concurrent valproate treatment (Messenheimer 2002). More recent data using a more gradual introduction indicate a much lower rate of serious rash in children (Messenheimer 2002). Due to its utility in adult bipolar depression (Calabrese et al. 1999) and maintenance treatment (Bowden et al. 2003; Calabrese et al. 2003), lamotrigine has begun to be studied in children and adolescents with bipolar disorder.

Twenty-three adolescents with bipolar I depression or mixed mania were evaluated in a 12-week, open-label study of lamotrigine monotherapy (Swope et al. 2004). Thirteen patients completed the study. Mean scores on the Montgomery-Åsberg Depression Rating Scale (MADRS) decreased from 21 at baseline to 4 at 12 weeks. Lamotrigine was reportedly well tolerated, with no incidence of rash or other adverse effect that caused discontinuation from the study. In another open prospective study, 20 adolescents with bipolar I, II, or NOS disorder in a depressive episode were treated with lamotrigine monotherapy or adjunct therapy for 8 weeks. The mean final dosage was 132 ± 31 mg/day, and 7 (37%) subjects were taking other mood stabilizers or atypical antipsychotics. Of 19 evaluable subjects, 16 (84%) were considered responders by Clinical Global Impression–Improvement (CGI-I; score of 1 or 2), and 12 (63%) responded by secondary criteria (at least a 50% decrease in CDRS-R scores) (Chang et al. 2005). Subjects with a baseline Young Mania Rating Scale (YMRS) score greater than 20 were less likely to be responders by secondary criteria. Children's Depression Rating Scale–Revised scores decreased significantly from baseline to the end of the study (mean change=−30.1±11.9). Lamotrigine was overall well tolerated, with reported adverse effects including headache (84%), slight fatigue (58%), nausea (53%), and increased perspiration (47%). No subject discontinued the study due to adverse effects, and there were no serious rashes. Furthermore, there was no significant change in weight over the course of the study, with a mean change of 0.42 ± 1.9 kg. In a retrospective chart review, Carandang et al. (2003) reported on nine adolescents with treatment-refractory mood disorders (six with bipolar depression) in whom lamotrigine was used as mono- or adjunctive therapy. At a mean daily dosage of 141.7 mg, improvement was noted in eight patients on the Clinical Global Impression (CGI) Scale for bipolar illness. One patient did develop a erythematous rash that resolved after medication was discontinued. These reports support the further study of this compound in pediatric bipolar disorder.

Topiramate

Open-label topiramate has been reported effective in pediatric bipolar disorder. DelBello and colleagues (2002) conducted a retrospective chart review of 26 children and adolescents (mean age 14±3.5 years) with bipolar I or II disorder, including 13 with comorbid ADHD. Subjects were treated with adjunctive or monotherapy topiramate for 1–30 months (mean 4.1±6.1 months). Seventy-three percent reported significant improvement in manic symptoms, 62% had overall improvement in psychiatric illness, and 38% had decreased ADHD symptom severity. Dosages ranged from 25 mg/day to 400 mg/day (mean 104±77 mg/day), and there were no serious adverse events.

A recent 4-week placebo-controlled topiramate trial (mean final dosage 278 mg/day) in 56 children and adolescents with bipolar I disorder (ages 6–17) with acute pure or mixed mania suggested efficacy, particularly for mixed mania (DelBello 2003). CGI-I scores at day 28 of treatment for completers were significantly better with topiramate compared with placebo. As noted in Chapter 2, controlled trials in adults have not been encouraging.

Topiramate has been generally well tolerated in children and adolescents. Most adverse events are mild to moderate and involve working memory problems, renal calculi, or weight loss. The latter is a potentially beneficial effect for patients experiencing weight gain while taking other mood stabilizers.

Other Novel Anticonvulsants

In one case report, oxcarbazepine added to lithium improved symptoms in a 6-year-old girl diagnosed with bipolar I disorder (Teitelbaum 2001). In one controlled clinical trial in pediatric epilepsy, 91% of children treated with adjunct oxcarbazepine (mean dosage 31.4 mg/kg/day) and 82% of subjects taking placebo experienced mild to moderate adverse events (Glauser et al. 2000). Adverse reactions were usually associated with the central nervous system (somnolence, dizziness) and the digestive system (nausea, vomiting). Finally, Davanzo and colleagues (Davanzo et al. 2004) reported on two boys with bipolar disorder, aged 12 and 15 years, successfully treated with adjunct oxcarbazepine at 900 mg and 450 mg/day respectively. Neither patient reported any adverse effects.

There are no data regarding the use of levetiracetam or tiagabine in pediatric bipolar disorder. However, levetiracetam has a generally well-tolerated safety profile in epilepsy treatment. In a study of 24 pediatric epilepsy patients, five reported adverse events such as diarrhea, lethargy, decreased appetite, and dizziness (Pellock et al. 2001). A study of epilepsy treatment in children taking tiagabine reported the most common adverse reactions to be asthenia, nervousness, dizziness, and somnolence (Uldall et al. 2000). However, efficacy and tolerability concerns have been raised regarding tiagabine in adults, with the latter including treatment-emergent seizures in bipolar disorder patients with no history of epilepsy (Grunze et al. 1999; Suppes et al. 2002). Despite no strong evidence for efficacy in adult mania of either agent, further studies of levetiracetam and, to a lesser degree, tiagabine in pediatric bipolar disorder ought to be considered given the tolerability profile and developmental differences between children and adults.

Atypical Antipsychotics

Atypical antipsychotic medications have had a substantial impact on pediatric psychopharmacology due to the presence of fewer adverse effects such as tardive dyskinesia, but they have not been studied as well as lithium and divalproex. There is a substantial amount of controlled research with atypical antipsychotics in adults for acute mania, acute bipolar depression, and maintenance therapy, as described in Chapters 2, 3, and 4, respectively, in this volume. In contrast, there are no published double-blind, placebo-controlled studies to date examining atypical antipsychotics as monotherapy for childhood bipolar disorder. However, case reports, retrospective case series, and prospective open-label studies suggest efficacy in pediatric mania.

Clozapine

Clozapine has been found useful in treatment-refractory pediatric bipolar disorder in a few case reports (Kowatch et al. 1995) and one open case series (Masi et al. 2002). In the latter report, 10 adolescents (12–17 years of age) with acute manic or mixed episodes who had failed to respond to standard treatment were treated with clozapine as monotherapy or adjunctive to lithium or valproate. All subjects responded based on the CGI-Improvement Scale. Mean effective dosage was 142.5 mg/day (75–300 mg/day) and main adverse effects were weight gain (7.0 kg over 6 months) and sedation. There were no significant decreases in white blood cell counts.

Olanzapine

Although the FDA has approved olanzapine for the treatment of mania in adults with bipolar disorders, this medication has been investigated only to a limited extent in pediatric bipolar disorder. Open data suggest olanzapine may be effective in mania in children and adolescents. In an outpatient case series of three prepubertal children with bipolar disorder, Chang and Ketter (2000) reported decreased manic symptoms in all patients within 3–5 days of administering olanzapine in conjunction with another mood stabilizer. In another open case series, five of seven adolescents with mania responded either to the addition of olanzapine to their medication regimens or, in one case, to olanzapine monotherapy (Soutullo et al. 1999). The predominant adverse effects for both reports were sedation and weight gain. In an 8-week prospective trial in 23 youth ages 5–14 years with bipolar disorder (mean, 10.3 years) (Frazier et al. 2001), open olanzapine monotherapy at a mean dosage of 9.6 mg/day yielded significant improvement in 61% of subjects. The most frequently reported adverse effects were increase in appetite, somnolence, abdominal pain, mild prolactin elevations, and a statistically significant increase in weight (5.0±2.3 kg). Controlled trials are needed to determine whether olanzapine may be effective for the treatment of acute mania in youth. Although the FDA has approved olanzapine as maintenance treatment and the combination of olanzapine and fluoxetine for the treatment of bipolar depression in adults with bipolar disorders, data are lacking regarding these uses in children and adolescents with bipolar disorder.

Quetiapine

Again, despite receiving FDA approval for the treatment of mania in adults with bipolar disorders, quetiapine has been investigated only moderately in pediatric bipolar disorder. Three adolescents with psychotic mania were reported to respond well to quetiapine monotherapy (McConville et al. 2000) acutely (mean dosage 600 mg/day) and over 88 weeks (McConville et al. 2003). There were no adverse effects such as extrapyramidal symptoms. Mean body mass index increased by 1.3 over 64 weeks. The most common adverse events were somnolence, headache, and pharyngitis.

In a rare double-blind, double-dummy study, DelBello and colleagues (2004) compared quetiapine to divalproex monotherapy in 50 acutely manic or mixed adolescent inpatients (mean age 15±2 years). Quetiapine dosage was begun at 100 mg/day and increased each day by 100 mg to a target dosage of 400 mg/day (mean final daily dose=415 mg). Patients were treated over 4 weeks. Response, considered a CGI-I score of 2 or less, was significantly higher for the quetiapine group (84%) than for the divalproex group (56%; $P=0.03$). Furthermore, more subjects achieved remission (less than 12 on the YMRS) in the quetiapine group compared to the divalproex group (60% versus 30% respectively). There were no group differences in adverse events, change in laboratory values, or change in extrapyramidal symptoms. Furthermore, change in weight over the study was not statistically different between the groups (divalproex=+3.6 kg, quetiapine=+4.4 kg). Because this was designed as a comparator study, the authors concluded that quetiapine was at least as efficacious as divalproex. These encouraging results suggest that further placebo-controlled studies with quetiapine monotherapy in adolescents and younger children with bipolar disorder should be conducted. Although quetiapine monotherapy has not yet been studied in a controlled fashion in pediatric bipolar disorder, there are data supporting its efficacy as an adjunct treatment (see "Combination Treatment" later in this chapter).

Risperidone

Similar to olanzapine and quetiapine, risperidone is approved by the FDA for the treatment of mania in adults with bipolar disorders yet has received little attention in pediatric bipolar disorder. Frazier et al. (1999) conducted a chart review of risperidone added to ongoing pharmacological treatments in youth with bipolar disorder ($N=28$, mean age 10.4±3.8). Addition of risperidone to ongoing medications yielded rapid, robust, and sustained responses for controlling manic (82%), psychotic (69%), and aggressive symptoms (82%). The main adverse effects were sedation and weight gain. Mean dosage of risperidone was 1.7 mg/day and mean duration of treatment was 6 months. These encouraging results indicate that prospective, controlled studies of this medication are warranted.

Ziprasidone and Aripiprazole

Although ziprasidone and aripiprazole have recently received FDA approval for the treatment of adults with bipolar disorder, no controlled trials have yet been conducted in children with bipolar disorder. Yet, there are some recent case reports and chart reviews published regarding the use of these agents in pediatric patients. Ziprasidone was reported effective in four children and adolescents, who had symptoms of mania and depression (Barnett 2004). However, while these children were diagnosed with bipolar disorder by the treating clinician, descriptions of the patients indicate that they may have better fit DSM-IV-TR criteria for bipolar disorder, not otherwise specified, schizoaffective disorder, bipolar type, or substance-induced mania (one patient had manic symptoms precipitated by paroxetine). Nonetheless, final ziprasidone dosages ranged from 40–80 mg/day, with adverse effects reported of sedation in two patients, and akathisia and tachycardia (with a normal QTc interval on ECG) in another.

A retrospective chart review of 30 children and adolescents with bipolar disorder or schizoaffective disorder, bipolar type, reported on the efficacy of aripiprazole in adjunct or monotherapy (Barzman et al. 2004). Patients presented with either mania, hypomania, depression, or mixed states, and most (87%) did not have psychotic symptoms. Mean starting dosage was 9±4 mg/day and mean final dosage was 10±3 mg/day. Treatment with aripiprazole lasted 1–9 months. Response, defined as a 1 or a 2 on a retrospectively determined CGI-I, was found in 67% of subjects. The most common adverse effects were sedation (33%), akathisia (23%), and gastrointestinal problems (7%). Of 14 subjects with weight data, 12 (86%) lost a mean of 3±6 kg. However, eight patients had experienced weight gain on other medications prior to the start of aripiprazole treatment.

Antipsychotic Drug Use in Bipolar Psychosis

It has not yet been unequivocally established whether treatment of psychosis in pediatric bipolar disorder requires antipsychotic medications. A systematic evaluation of lithium and adjunctive haloperidol (mean lithium dosage 1,560 mg/day; mean serum level 0.93 mEq/L) in five bipolar youth with psychotic features reported resolution of psychosis after 1 week, with symptom relapse after subsequent discontinuation of the haloperidol (Kafantaris et al. 2001b). The same authors conducted a similar open-label study in 42 adolescents (mean age 16 years) with acute mania with psychotic features (Kafantaris et al. 2001a). The adolescents received open treatment with lithium (mean serum concentration 0.89 mEq/mL) and haloperidol (53.6%, mean dosage 5 mg/day), risperidone (21.4%, mean dosage 2.25 mg/day), or another atypical antipsychotic. Significant improvement after 4 weeks of combination treatment was seen in 61% of subjects, who then tapered off the antipsychotic. However, within 1 week of antipsychotic discontinuation, 43% had relapse of aggression or psychosis necessitating antipsychotic reintroduction. Only 29% of patients were successfully treated with lithium monotherapy. These findings suggest that youth with psychotic mania may need antipsychotic treatment for more than 4 weeks.

Efficacy data for atypical antipsychotics in pediatric mania are emerging, but it is not yet clear whether they should be considered first-line treatment in these children. The dearth of evidence to support longitudinal or monotherapy use in this population highlights the need for randomized, double-blind, placebo-controlled studies. In addition, adverse effects such as sedation, weight gain, and other metabolic effects (as reported in adults) need to be more thoroughly investigated, particularly in long-term treatment. For example, there are concerns that children and adolescents treated with atypical antipsychotics may experience more relative weight gain than adults (Stigler et al. 2004), and serum glucose elevations in such children have been reported (Koller et al. 2003). Because of possible induction of type II diabetes in adults treated with atypical antipsychotics, additional care such as glucose monitoring should be used when using these medications for children with bipolar disorder.

Other Medications

Levothyroxine (T4) may be an underutilized adjunctive treatment in pediatric bipolar disorder. Clearly, T4 is required if a patient develops sustained lithium-induced hypothyroidism, which may occur in up to 24% of such treated children (Gracious et al. 2004). Even with normal thyroid-stimulating hormone (TSH) levels, if a patient with bipolar disorder is displaying rapid cycling and symptoms are refractory to current medications, it may be worthwhile to consider treatment with moderate to high-dosage T4 (0.075–0.14 mg/day). The long-term effects of such treatment are unclear. It has been suggested that to avoid adverse cardiac and bone density effects it may be important to keep patients euthyroid by free T4 level monitoring and to avoid over-suppression of endogenous TSH (Bartalena et al. 1996; Williams 1997). However, some longitudinal studies have reported no adverse effects of chronic T4 treatment on heart function (Radetti et al. 1995) or bone density (Saggese et al. 1996) in children. Interestingly, omega-3 fatty acids have received attention as possible treatments for pediatric and adult bipolar disorder, despite limited data (Stoll et al. 1999). Other treatments with promise, but understudied in children, include nimodipine (Davanzo et al. 1999) and electroconvulsive therapy (Hill et al. 1997).

Combination Treatment

It is apparent that as with adults, most children and adolescents with bipolar disorder require treatment with more than one psychotropic medication. A questionnaire study of parents in the Child and Adolescent Bipolar Foundation found that most of their children were being treated with at least three psychotropic agents (M. Hellander, personal communication, June 2003). In a study by Kowatch and colleagues (2003), after open treatment for 6 weeks with either lithium, divalproex, or carbamazepine monotherapy, 35 subjects were followed naturalistically. Of these, 58% required combination treatment for full stabilization of mood and improvement in functioning, with 34% requiring addition of a stimulant, 11% an antipsychotic, and 6% an antidepressant. Additionally, 80% reached euthymic mood on two mood stabilizers. Systematic evaluations of combination pharmacotherapy for all phases of bipolar disorder in youth are needed. Two other studies also highlight the potential greater response to combination treatment.

DelBello et al. (2002) examined the addition of quetiapine

versus placebo to divalproex in hospitalized manic adolescents with bipolar disorder in a 6-week, randomized, double-blind study ($N=30$; mean age 14 ± 2 years). Subjects were loaded with divalproex 20 mg/kg/day and either quetiapine or placebo was added. Over 6 weeks, both groups had significant improvement, but those given divalproex and quetiapine yielded significantly greater reduction in manic symptoms and a higher percentage of responders as determined by CGI-Change Scale and a 50% reduction in YMRS score (87% versus 53%). Final valproate serum levels were about 100 µg/mL and mean quetiapine dosage was 432 mg/day. The divalproex plus quetiapine group compared with the divalproex monotherapy group had more sedation (80% versus 33%) and weight gain (4.2 kg versus 2.5 kg).

In a sample of 139 children and adolescents, aged 5–17 years, with bipolar I and II disorder, only 9% failed to respond to a combination of open lithium and divalproex over 20 weeks (Findling et al. 2003). Furthermore, 47% reached remission, as defined by 4 consecutive weeks of low mania and depression ratings and adequate functioning. Mean dosages were 923 mg/day for lithium and 863 mg/day for divalproex. Valproate serum levels were similar in those who remitted and those who did not, but lithium levels were not (1.0 mEq/L versus 0.7 mEq/L). Among non-remitters (who were withdrawn from consideration for the second part of the study), 40% had noncompliance, 29% unstable mood, 25% lithium intolerance, and 6% divalproex intolerance. Weight gain was 0.3 kg/week over the first 8 weeks and 0.2 kg/week thereafter, for a mean total of 3.0 kg. In the second phase of the study, remitters were randomized to discontinue either lithium or divalproex. In this phase, 75% of subjects dropped out, primarily due to unstable mood, and among the completers, 49% relapsed. There were no significant differences between survival rates in the divalproex and lithium groups (Findling 2002).

These studies suggest that most children and adolescents with bipolar disorder require combinations of at least two agents (in these cases divalproex plus lithium or an atypical antipsychotic). Additional studies of different medication combinations, used in different phases of illness, are needed to inform clinical practice.

Treatment of Comorbid Conditions

Childhood-onset bipolar disorder is commonly associated with or preceded by disruptive behavioral disorders such as conduct disorder, ADHD, and/or oppositional defiant disorder (ODD). Researchers have reported that as many as 57%–94% of bipolar children and adolescents have comorbid ADHD (Faraone et al. 1997; Geller et al. 2000) and 12%–41% have comorbid conduct disorder (Biederman et al. 1999; Masi et al. 2003; Tillman et al. 2003). Anxiety disorders may also be common (Masi et al. 2001). Therefore, comprehensive treatment of children and adolescents with bipolar disorder commonly entails treating comorbid conditions.

Disruptive Behavioral Disorders

Due to the high comorbidity of ADHD with pediatric bipolar disorder, symptoms of ADHD should be assessed after stabilization of mood symptoms. Typical ADHD treatments, such as psychostimulants, may be added to mood stabilizing agents at that time to treat syndromal or residual symptoms of ADHD. There is some concern that stimulants may worsen or cause manic symptoms in children with bipolar disorder (DelBello et al. 2001; Soutullo et al. 2002), but there is currently equivocal evidence regarding this concern (Carlson and Kelly 2003; Galanter et al. 2003). One double-blind, controlled study found mixed salts amphetamine (mean dosage 14.5 ± 5.8 mg/day) added to divalproex (median dosage 750 mg/day, mean serum concentration 82.9 ± 14.4 µg/mL) to be superior to placebo for ADHD symptoms in children and adolescents with bipolar disorder and ADHD (Scheffer et al. 2005). One of 30 subjects had a manic episode attributable to the addition of amphetamine, which resolved upon discontinuation of the stimulant. Therefore, if treating comorbid ADHD with stimulants or atomoxetine after mood stabilization has been achieved, it is important to monitor closely for emergence of manic symptoms (Chang and DelBello 2003).

There are no data regarding medications for comorbid ODD in pediatric bipolar disorder. Symptoms of ODD may improve after mood stabilization. Similarly, although there have been no studies specifically concerning treatment of conduct disorder comorbid with pediatric bipolar disorder, agents that are effective in pediatric mania may also improve symptoms of aggression and conduct disorder (Steiner et al. 2003a, 2003b).

Anxiety Disorders

Pharmacological treatment of comorbid anxiety may be challenging due to 1) the tendency to use selective serotonin reuptake inhibitors (SSRIs) for anxiety disorders and 2) the possibility of destabilizing mood with SSRIs in children and adolescents with bipolar disorder (Chang et al. 2001; Faedda et al. 2004). Current treatments should therefore focus on nonpharmacological interventions such as cognitive-behavioral therapy or cautious use of SSRIs in these children. Another possibility is the adjunctive use of gabapentin, given its efficacy in social phobia and panic disorder in adults (Pande et al. 1999, 2000b) and probable low propensity for mood destabilization (Pande et al. 2000a). However, as noted earlier, gabapentin has been associated with behavioral toxicity in children with epilepsy. No studies have examined the use of benzodiazepines in children with bipolar disorder and anxiety. However, given potential complications of tolerance, addiction, and treatment-emergent mania (Freeman et al. 2002) and reports of behavioral disinhibition in children (Graae et al. 1994), benzodiazepines should only be used second-line and cautiously in this population. Other suitable treatments for comorbid anxiety in pediatric bipolar disorder need to be studied.

Substance Abuse

There are few specific prospective studies of treating comorbid substance abuse in this population. In the previously mentioned study by Geller et al. (1998), lithium was superior to placebo in reducing positive toxicology screens in adolescents with bipolar disorder. Therefore, studies of mood stabilizers to treat mania as well as decrease substance use in pediatric bipolar disorder are warranted.

Acute Bipolar Depression

Emerging controlled data regarding the management of acute bipolar depression are described in Chapter 3 in this volume. Although the treatment of acute bipolar depression in pediatric populations has not been studied, it warrants a special mention here because SSRIs may be particularly problematic when treating children with bipolar disorder. As in adults, there have been numerous reports of SSRI-induced mania in children and adolescents (Chang et al. 2001), most of whom were treated for depression or anxiety. Less clear is whether SSRIs can be acutely or gradually destabilizing in pediatric bipolar disorder. There have been concerns, originally raised by from European and United States regulatory agencies and academics, that SSRIs may cause suicidal behavior in some children. This idea originated from data from pediatric clinical trials of SSRIs, shared with the United Kingdom and United States regulatory agencies by pharmaceutical companies, that revealed a higher incidence of "suicidal behaviors" occurring with SSRIs compared with placebo in participating subjects (Abbott 2003; Mitka 2003). Because depression is often the first presenting mood episode in patients with bipolar disorder (Lish et al. 1994), it is possible that many of these presumed unipolar depressed children actually were experiencing an initial bipolar depressive episode. Because SSRIs may cause or exacerbate mania in adults with bipolar disorder (Post et al. 2003), these children may have experienced manic or mixed symptoms leading to greater suicidality and impulsivity. Until further data are obtained on this issue, caution is recommended when utilizing SSRIs in pediatric patients with bipolar disorder.

Psychotherapy

Emerging data suggest that children and adolescents can benefit from psychotherapy. Two interventions with evidence of efficacy in adult patients with bipolar disorder are cognitive therapy (Lam et al. 2003) and family-focused therapy (Miklowitz et al. 2000; Rea et al. 2003). Miklowitz et al. (2004) investigated the efficacy of family-focused therapy in 20 adolescents with bipolar disorder (mean age 14.8 years). The treatment included 21 sessions over 9 months as well as optional continuation sessions every 3 months. Thereafter participants received manualized psychoeducation, communication enhancement training, and problem-solving skills training. Improvements in manic and depressive symptoms and behavior problems were seen at 1-year follow-up. Further studies investigating the use of these approaches in children and adolescents are currently in progress.

Adjunctive psychoeducation has also been examined in pediatric bipolar disorder. A recent study investigated multifamily psychoeducation groups for mood-disordered children (ages 8–11) and their families (Fristad et al. 2002, 2003a). Treatment consisted of eight 90-minute sessions in which parents and children from different families met together and separately to learn about the illness and its treatment. Sessions included communication exercises, cognitive-behavioral interventions, and problem-solving skills training, focusing on the children's mood symptom management. At 6-month follow-up, this approach was associated with increased parental knowledge about children's mood symptoms, increased positive family interactions, and increased perception of parental support as reported by the children (Fristad et al. 2003b).

Lifecharting (Denicoff et al. 1997; Leverich et al. 1990) may help adolescents identify their moods and precipitants of manic or depressive episodes. Although adolescents may have difficulties with such "homework," parents can be encouraged to work with their children to keep an ongoing record of mood variations, stressors, sleep, and medication.

The practical and family-focused therapies just described appear to be valuable adjuncts to medications for treating children and adolescents with bipolar disorder. More research is needed in this area, particularly regarding psychiatric treatment of bipolar depression in adolescents, given the safety and efficacy concerns regarding the use of antidepressant medication in this population and encouraging data regarding psychotherapy for adolescents with unipolar depression (Mufson et al. 2004).

Prevention

Ultimately, efforts need to be made in preventing the onset of bipolar disorder in children and adolescents. Although children at high risk for developing bipolar disorder are beginning to be characterized (Chang et al. 2003c), studies are needed to determine which children are most appropriate for early intervention and what treatment modalities (medications or psychotherapies) ought to be used. Nevertheless, researchers have begun to generate hypotheses regarding these issues, and it is hoped that this field will ultimately progress to provide guidelines for early intervention and prevention of bipolar disorder.

Assuming children with prodromal bipolar disorder can be identified (Chang et al. 2003b), there are a few strategies that could be employed for early intervention and prevention. Pharmacological or psychotherapeutic approaches could be instituted to prevent, delay, or attenuate bipolar disorder development. As hypothesized by the kindling model, the illness development and/or progression could be avoided, haltered, or even reversed by appropriate medications. Pharmacology could prevent the progression of bipolar disorder by initially and appropriately treating putative prodromal symptoms such as ADHD and mood symptoms. Then, by preventing future mood episodes and/or through intrinsic neuroprotective properties, interventions could potentially prevent the development of full bipolar disorder. Medications already being used to treat pediatric bipolar disorder may be promising candidates for early intervention due to the neuroprotective qualities of lithium and certain anticonvulsants (Manji and Chen 2002; Manji et al. 2000). In an early study with relevance to the pharmacological prevention model, Chang et al. (2003a) investigated the use of divalproex monotherapy in 24 bipolar offspring with mood and/or disruptive behavioral disorders. None of the subjects, aged 7–17, had bipolar I or II disorder, but all had at least some mild affective symptoms as manifested by a minimum score of 12 on the YMRS or Hamilton Rating Scale for Depression. After 12 weeks of open divalproex monotherapy (mean dosage 821 mg/day, mean serum concentration 79.0 ± 26.8 µg/mL), 78% responded, with the majority showing improvement by week 3. Although this study demonstrated the potential of divalproex in putative prodromal bipolar disorder, longitudinal controlled studies are needed to determine the efficacy of such agents in actual prevention of bipolar disorder development.

Psychotherapeutic interventions could also prove useful for

early intervention. However, group cognitive therapy was no more effective than no specific intervention in reducing depressive symptoms of adolescent offspring of depressed parents (Clarke et al. 2002). Therefore, other more intensive modalities, such as family-focused therapy, may be needed for children at high risk for bipolar disorder development and could importantly complement pharmacological intervention studies.

Further research is needed to assess whether children at risk for bipolar disorder can be reliably identified before the onset of the first manic episode and whether interventions can successfully treat these children and prevent eventual fully developed bipolar disorder.

Conclusions

Research into the treatment of pediatric bipolar disorder has begun to offer substantial data from which treatment recommendations can eventually evolve. With the increased funding and mandated regulations from the United States government and other agencies to study the efficacy and safety of psychotropic medications in children and adolescents, it is likely that the gaps in data presented here will begin to be addressed. However, new compounds will continue to be developed for the treatment of bipolar disorder and will require separate study in pediatric populations. Furthermore, whereas acute mania has received more attention, other important areas, such as acute bipolar depression and maintenance therapy are only beginning to be adequately explored. Although not addressed here, educational interventions also are usually needed, due to the interference of the disorder and medications with normal schooling, and are essential to any treatment program for youth with bipolar disorder. Finally, psychotherapies should ideally be studied as adjunctive interventions in pediatric bipolar disorder. Extension of the evolving research described in this chapter will help advance the eventual goal of eradication of bipolar symptoms and perhaps ultimately permit prevention of bipolar disorder in children and adolescents at risk.

References

Abbott A: British panel bans use of antidepressant to treat children. Nature 423:792, 2003

American Psychiatric Association: Practice guideline for the treatment of patients with bipolar disorder (revision). Am J Psychiatry 159(suppl):1–50, 2002

Barnett, MS: Ziprasidone monotherapy in pediatric bipolar disorder. J Child Adolesc Psychopharmacol 14:471–477, 2004

Bartalena L, Bogazzi F, Martino E: Adverse effects of thyroid hormone preparations and antithyroid drugs. Drug Saf 15:53–63, 1996

Barzman DH, DelBello MP, Kowatch RA: The effectiveness and tolerability of ariprazole for pediatric bipolar disorders: a retrospective chart review. J Child Adolesc Psychopharmacol 14:593–600, 2004

Biederman J, Faraone SV, Chu MP, et al: Further evidence of a bidirectional overlap between juvenile mania and conduct disorder in children. J Am Acad Child Adolesc Psychiatry 38:468–476, 1999

Bowden CL, Calabrese JR, Sachs G, et al: A placebo-controlled 18-month trial of lamotrigine and lithium maintenance treatment in recently manic or hypomanic patients with bipolar I disorder. Arch Gen Psychiatry 60:392–400, 2003

Calabrese JR, Rapport DJ, Kimmel SE, et al: Rapid cycling bipolar disorder and its treatment with valproate. Can J Psychiatry 38 (suppl 2):S57–S61, 1993

Calabrese JR, Bowden CL, Sachs GS, et al: A double-blind placebo-controlled study of lamotrigine monotherapy in outpatients with bipolar I depression: Lamictal 602 Study Group. J Clin Psychiatry 60:79–88, 1999

Calabrese JR, Bowden CL, Sachs G, et al: A placebo-controlled 18-month trial of lamotrigine and lithium maintenance treatment in recently depressed patients with bipolar I disorder. J Clin Psychiatry 64:1013–1024, 2003

Carandang CG, Maxwell DJ, Robbins DR, et al: Lamotrigine in adolescent mood disorders. J Am Acad Child Adolesc Psychiatry 42:750–751, 2003

Carlson GA, Kelly KL: Stimulant rebound: how common is it and what does it mean? J Child Adolesc Psychopharmacol 13:137–142, 2003

Chang KD, DelBello MP: Stimulant use in pediatric bipolar disorder with attention-deficit/hyperactivity disorder. The Journal of Bipolar Disorders: Reviews and Commentaries II:3–17, 2003

Chang KD, Ketter TA: Mood stabilizer augmentation with olanzapine in acutely manic children. J Child Adolesc Psychopharmacol 10:45–49, 2000

Chang KD, Ketter TA: Special issues in the treatment of paediatric bipolar disorder. Expert Opin Pharmacother 2:613–622, 2001

Chang KD, Soutullo CS, Steiner H, et al: SSRI-induced mania In children and adolescents. Psychiatric Networks 4:55–63, 2001

Chang KD, Dienes K, Blasey C, et al: Divalproex monotherapy in the treatment of bipolar offspring with mood and behavioral disorders and at least mild affective symptoms. J Clin Psychiatry 64:936–942, 2003a

Chang K, Steiner H, Dienes K, et al: Bipolar offspring: a window into bipolar disorder evolution. Biol Psychiatry 53:945–551, 2003b

Chang K, Steiner H, Ketter T: Studies of offspring of parents with bipolar disorder. Am J Med Genet 123C:26–35, 2003c

Chang K, Saxena K, Howe M: Lamotrigine adjunctive or monotherapy in adolescent bipolar depression. Paper presented at the annual meeting of the American Psychiatric Association, Atlanta, GA, May 2005

Clarke GN, Hornbrook M, Lynch F, et al: Group cognitive-behavioral treatment for depressed adolescent offspring of depressed parents in a health maintenance organization. J Am Acad Child Adolesc Psychiatry 41:305–313, 2002

Davanzo PA, Krah N, Kleiner J, et al: Nimodipine treatment of an adolescent with ultradian cycling bipolar affective illness. J Child Adolesc Psychopharmacol 9:51–61, 1999

Davanzo PA, McCracken JT: Mood stabilizers in the treatment of juvenile bipolar disorder: advances and controversies. Child Adolesc Psychiatr Clin N Am 9:159–182, 2000

Davanzo PA, Nikore V, Yehya N, et al: Oxcarbazepine treatment of juvenile-onset bipolar disorder. J Child Adolesc Psychopharmacol 14:344–345, 2004

DelBello MP, Kowatch RA, Warner J, et al: Adjunctive topiramate treatment for pediatric bipolar disorder: a restrospective chart review. J Child Adolesc Psychopharmacol 12:323–330, 2002

DelBello MP: Topiramate treatment for acute mania in children and adolescents with bipolar I disorder. Presented at the 42nd annual meeting of the American College of Neuropsychopharmacology, San Juan, Puerto Rico, December 2003

DelBello MP, Soutullo CA, Hendricks W, et al: Prior stimulant treatment in adolescents with bipolar disorder: association with age at onset. Bipolar Disord 3:53–57, 2001

DelBello MP, Schwiers ML, Rosenberg HL, et al: A double-blind, randomized, placebo-controlled study of quetiapine as adjunctive treatment for adolescent mania. J Am Acad Child Adolesc Psychiatry 41:1216–1223, 2002

DelBello MP, Kowatch RA, Adler C, et al: A double-blind comparison of divalproex versus quetiapine for adolescent mania. Paper presented at the annual meeting of the American Academy of Child and Adolescent Psychiatry, Washington, DC, October 2004

DeLong GR: Lithium carbonate treatment of select behavior disorders in children suggesting manic-depressive illness. J Pediatr 93:689–694, 1978

Denicoff KD, Smith-Jackson EE, Disney ER, et al: Preliminary evidence of the reliability and validity of the prospective life-chart methodology (LCM-p). J Psychiatr Res 31:593–603, 1997

Dooley J, Camfield P, Gordon K, et al: Lamotrigine-induced rash in children. Neurology 46:240–242, 1996

Faraone SV, Biederman J, Wozniak J, et al: Is comorbidity with ADHD a marker for juvenile-onset mania? J Am Acad Child Adolesc Psychiatry 36:1046–1055, 1997

Faedda GL, Baldessarini RJ, Glovinsky IP, et al: Treatment-emergent mania in pediatric bipolar disorder: a retrospective case review. J Affect Disord 82:149–158, 2004

Findling RL: Combination pharmacotherapy in pediatric bipolar disorders, in Scientific Proceedings of the 49th Annual Meeting of the American Academy of Child and Adolescent Psychiatry. San Francisco, CA, October, 2002, p 33

Findling RL, Gracious BL, McNamara NK, et al: Rapid, continuous cycling and psychiatric co-morbidity in pediatric bipolar I disorder. Bipolar Disord 3:202–210, 2001

Findling RL, McNamara NK, Gracious BL, et al: Combination lithium and divalproex sodium in pediatric bipolarity. J Am Acad Child Adolesc Psychiatry 42:895–901, 2003

Frazier JA, Meyer MC, Biederman J, et al: Risperidone treatment for juvenile bipolar disorder: a retrospective chart review. J Am Acad Child Adolesc Psychiatry 38:960–965, 1999

Frazier JA, Biederman J, Tohen M, et al: A prospective open-label treatment trial of olanzapine monotherapy in children and adolescents with bipolar disorder. J Child Adolesc Psychopharmacol 11:239–250, 2001

Freeman MP, Freeman SA, McElroy SL: The comorbidity of bipolar and anxiety disorders: prevalence, psychobiology, and treatment issues. J Affect Disord 68:1–23, 2002

Fristad MA, Goldberg-Arnold JS, Gavazzi SM: Multifamily psychoeducation groups (MFPG) for families of children with bipolar disorder. Bipolar Disord 4:254–262, 2002

Fristad MA, Gavazzi SM, Mackinaw-Koons B: Family psychoeducation: an adjunctive intervention for children with bipolar disorder. Biol Psychiatry 53:1000–1008, 2003a

Fristad MA, Goldberg-Arnold JS, Gavazzi SM: Multi-family psychoeducation groups in the treatment of children with mood disorders. J Marital Fam Ther 29:491–504, 2003b

Galanter CA, Carlson GA, Jensen PS, et al: Response to methylphenidate in children with attention deficit hyperactivity disorder and manic symptoms in the multimodal treatment study of children with attention deficit hyperactivity disorder titration trial. J Child Adolesc Psychopharmacol 13:123–136, 2003

Geller B, Sun K, Zimerman B, et al: Complex and rapid-cycling in bipolar children and adolescents: a preliminary study. J Affect Disord 34:259–268, 1995

Geller B, Cooper TB, Sun K, et al: Double-blind and placebo-controlled study of lithium for adolescent bipolar disorders with secondary substance dependency. J Am Acad Child Adolesc Psychiatry 37:171–178, 1998

Geller B, Zimerman B, Williams M, et al: Diagnostic characteristics of 93 cases of a prepubertal and early adolescent bipolar disorder phenotype by gender, puberty and comorbid attention deficit hyperactivity disorder. J Child Adolesc Psychopharmacol 10:157–164, 2000

Geller B, Craney JL, Bolhofner K, et al: Two-year prospective follow-up of children with a prepubertal and early adolescent bipolar disorder phenotype. Am J Psychiatry 159:927–933, 2002

Glauser TA, Nigro M, Sachdeo R, et al: Adjunctive therapy with oxcarbazepine in children with partial seizures: The Oxcarbazepine Pediatric Study Group. Neurology 54:2237–2244, 2000

Graae F, Milner J, Rizzotto L, et al: Clonazepam in childhood anxiety disorders. J Am Acad Child Adolesc Psychiatry 33:372–376, 1994

Gracious BL, Findling RL, Seman C, et al: Elevated thyrotropin in bipolar youths prescribed both lithium and divalproex sodium. J Am Acad Child Adolesc Psychiatry 43:215–220, 2004

Grunze H, Erfurth A, Marcuse A, et al: Tiagabine appears not to be efficacious in the treatment of acute mania. J Clin Psychiatry 60:759–762, 1999

Hamrin V, Bailey K: Gabapentin and methylphenidate treatment of a preadolescent with attention deficit hyperactivity disorder and bipolar disorder. J Child Adolesc Psychopharmacol 11:301–309, 2001

Hassanyeh F, Davison K: Bipolar affective psychosis with onset before age 16 years: report of 10 cases. Br J Psychiatry 137:530–539, 1980

Henry CA, Zamvil LS, Lam C, et al: Long-term outcome with divalproex in children and adolescents with bipolar disorder. J Child Adolesc Psychopharmacol 13:523–529, 2003

Hill MA, Courvoisie H, Dawkins K, et al: ECT for the treatment of intractable mania in two prepubertal male children. Convuls Ther 13:74–82, 1997

Himmelhoch JM, Garfinkel ME: Sources of lithium resistance in mixed mania. Psychopharmacol Bull 22:613–620, 1986

Hsu LK: Lithium-resistant adolescent mania. J Am Acad Child Psychiatry 25:280–283, 1986

Kafantaris V, Coletti DJ, Dicker R, et al: Adjunctive antipsychotic treatment of adolescents with bipolar psychosis. J Am Acad Child Adolesc Psychiatry 40:1448–1456, 2001a

Kafantaris V, Dicker R, Coletti DJ, et al: Adjunctive antipsychotic treatment is necessary for adolescents with psychotic mania. J Child Adolesc Psychopharmacol 11:409–413, 2001b

Kafantaris V, Coletti DJ, Dicker R, et al: Lithium treatment of acute mania in adolescents: a large open trial. J Am Acad Child Adolesc Psychiatry 42:1038–1045, 2003

Keck PE Jr, Perlis RH, Otto MW, et al: The expert consensus guideline series: treatment of bipolar disorder 2004. Postgrad Med (Spec):1–20, 2004

Khurana DS, Riviello J, Helmers S, et al: Efficacy of gabapentin therapy in children with refractory partial seizures. J Pediatr 128:829–833, 1996

Koller EA, Cross JT, Doraiswamy PM, et al: Risperidone-associated diabetes mellitus: a pharmacovigilance study. Pharmacotherapy 23:735–744, 2003

Kowatch RA, DelBello MP: The use of mood stabilizers and atypical antipsychotics in children and adolescents with bipolar disorders. CNS Spectr 8:273–280, 2003

Kowatch RA, Sethuraman G, Hume JH, et al: Combination pharmacotherapy in children and adolescents with bipolar disorder. Biol Psychiatry 53:978–984, 2003

Kowatch R, Suppes T, Gilfillan SK, et al: Clozapine treatment of children and adolescents with bipolar disorder and schizophrenia: a clinical case series. J Child Adolesc Psychopharmacol 5:241–253, 1995

Kowatch RA, Suppes T, Carmody TJ, et al: Effect size of lithium, divalproex sodium, and carbamazepine in children and adolescents with bipolar disorder. J Am Acad Child Adolesc Psychiatry 39:713–720, 2000

Kusumakar V, Yatham LN: An open study of lamotrigine in refractory bipolar depression. Psychiatry Res 72:145–148, 1997

Kutcher SP, Marton P, Korenblum M: Adolescent bipolar illness and personality disorder. J Am Acad Child Adolesc Psychiatry 29:355–358, 1990

Lam DH, Watkins ER, Hayward P, et al: A randomized controlled study of cognitive therapy for relapse prevention for bipolar affective disorder: outcome of the first year. Arch Gen Psychiatry 60:145–152, 2003

Lee DO, Steingard RJ, Cesena M, et al: Behavioral side effects of gabapentin in children. Epilepsia 37:87–90, 1996

Leverich GS, Post RM, Rosoff AS: Factors associated with relapse during maintenance treatment of affective disorders. Int Clin Psychopharmacol 5:135–156, 1990

Lish JD, Dime-Meenan S, Whybrow PC, et al: National Depressive and Manic-Depressive Association (DMDA) survey of bipolar members. J Affect Disord 31:281–294, 1994

Manji HK, Chen G: PKC, MAP kinases and the bcl-2 family of proteins as long-term targets for mood stabilizers. Mol Psychiatry 7 (suppl 1):S46–S56, 2002

Manji HK, Moore GJ, Chen G: Clinical and preclinical evidence for the neurotrophic effects of mood stabilizers: implications for the pathophysiology and treatment of manic-depressive illness. Biol Psychiatry 48:740–754, 2000

Masi G, Toni C, Perugi G, et al: Anxiety disorders in children and adolescents with bipolar disorder: a neglected comorbidity. Can J Psychiatry 46:797–802, 2001

Masi G, Mucci M, Millepiedi S: Clozapine in adolescent inpatients with acute mania. J Child Adolesc Psychopharmacol 12:93–99, 2002

Masi G, Toni C, Perugi G, et al: Externalizing disorders in consecutively referred children and adolescents with bipolar disorder. Compr Psychiatry 44:184–189, 2003

McConville BJ, Arvanitis LA, Thyrum PT, et al: Pharmacokinetics, tolerability, and clinical effectiveness of quetiapine fumarate: an open-label trial in adolescents with psychotic disorders. J Clin Psychiatry 61:252–260, 2000

McConville B, Carrero L, Sweitzer D, et al: Long-term safety, tolerability, and clinical efficacy of quetiapine in adolescents: an open-label extension trial. J Child Adolesc Psychopharmacol 13:75–82, 2003

McKnew DH, Cytryn L, Buchsbaum MS, et al: Lithium in children of lithium-responding parents. Psychiatry Res 4:171–180, 1981

McLean MJ: Gabapentin. Epilepsia 36 (suppl 2):S73–S86, 1995

Messenheimer J: Efficacy and safety of lamotrigine in pediatric patients. J Child Neurol 17 (suppl 2):2S34–2S42, 2002

Messenheimer JA, Giorgi L, Risner ME: The tolerability of lamotrigine in children. Drug Saf 22:303–312, 2000

Miklowitz DJ, Simoneau TL, George EL, et al: Family focused treatment of bipolar disorder: 1-year effects of a psychoeducational program in conjunction with pharmacotherapy. Biol Psychiatry 48:582–592, 2000

Miklowitz DJ, George EL, Axelson DA, et al: Family-focused treatment for adolescents with bipolar disorder. J Affect Disord 82 (suppl 1):S113–128, 2004

Mitka M: FDA alert on antidepressants for youth. JAMA 290:2534, 2003

Mota-Castillo M, Torruella A, Engels B, et al: Valproate in very young children: an open case series with a brief follow-up. J Affect Disord 67:193–197, 2001

Mufson L, Dorta KP, Wickramaratne P, et al: A randomized effectiveness trial of interpersonal psychotherapy for depressed adolescents. Arch Gen Psychiatry 61:577–584, 2004

Pande AC, Davidson JR, Jefferson JW, et al: Treatment of social phobia with gabapentin: a placebo-controlled study. J Clin Psychopharmacol 19:341–348, 1999

Pande AC, Crockatt JG, Janney CA, et al: Gabapentin in bipolar disorder: a placebo-controlled trial of adjunctive therapy: Gabapentin Bipolar Disorder Study Group. Bipolar Disord 2:249–255, 2000a

Pande AC, Pollack MH, Crockatt J, et al: Placebo-controlled study of gabapentin treatment of panic disorder. J Clin Psychopharmacol 20:467–471, 2000b

Papatheodorou G, Kutcher SP: Divalproex sodium treatment in late adolescent and young adult acute mania. Psychopharmacol Bull 29:213–219, 1993

Papatheodorou G, Kutcher SP, Katic M, et al: The efficacy and safety of divalproex sodium in the treatment of acute mania in adolescents and young adults: an open clinical trial. J Clin Psychopharmacol 15:110–116, 1995

Pellock JM, Glauser TA, Bebin EM, et al: Pharmacokinetic study of levetiracetam in children. Epilepsia 42:1574–1579, 2001

Post RM, Leverich GS, Nolen WA, et al: A re-evaluation of the role of antidepressants in the treatment of bipolar depression: data from the Stanley Foundation Bipolar Network. Bipolar Disord 5:396–406, 2003

Radetti G, Paganini C, Crepaz R, et al: Cardiovascular effects of long-term L-thyroxine therapy for Hashimoto's thyroiditis in children and adolescents. Eur J Endocrinol 132:688–692, 1995

Rea MM, Tompson MC, Miklowitz DJ, et al: Family focused treatment versus individual treatment for bipolar disorder: results of a randomized clinical trial. J Consult Clin Psychol 71:482–492, 2003

Saggese G, Bertelloni S, Baroncelli GI, et al: Bone mineral density in adolescent females treated with L-thyroxine: a longitudinal study. Eur J Pediatr 155:452–457, 1996

Schaeffer R, Kowatch R, Carmody T, et al: Randomized, placebo-controlled trial of mixed aphetamine salts for symptoms of comorbid ADHD in pediatric bipolar disorder after mood stabilization with divalproex sodium. Am J Psychiatry 162:58–64, 2005

Soutullo CA, Casuto LS, Keck PE Jr: Gabapentin in the treatment of adolescent mania: a case report. J Child Adolesc Psychopharmacol 8:81–85, 1998

Soutullo CA, Sorter MT, Foster KD, et al: Olanzapine in the treatment of adolescent acute mania: a report of seven cases. J Affect Disord 53:279–283, 1999

Soutullo CA, DelBello MP, Ochsner JE, et al: Severity of bipolarity in hospitalized manic adolescents with history of stimulant or antidepressant treatment. J Affect Disord 70:323–327, 2002

Steiner H, Petersen ML, Saxena K, et al: Divalproex sodium for the treatment of conduct disorder: a randomized controlled clinical trial. J Clin Psychiatry 64:1183–1191, 2003a

Steiner H, Saxena K, Chang K: Psychopharmacologic strategies for the treatment of aggression in juveniles. CNS Spectr 8:298–308, 2003b

Stigler KA, Potenza MN, Posey DJ, et al: Weight gain associated with atypical antipsychotic use in children and adolescents: prevalence, clinical relevance, and management. Paediatr Drugs 6:33–44, 2004

Stoll AL, Severus WE, Freeman MP, et al: Omega 3 fatty acids in bipolar disorder: a preliminary double-blind, placebo-controlled trial. Arch Gen Psychiatry 56:407–412, 1999

Strober M, Morrell W, Burroughs J, et al: A family study of bipolar I disorder in adolescence: early onset of symptoms linked to increased familial loading and lithium resistance. J Affect Disord 15:255–268, 1988

Strober M, Morrell W, Lampert C, et al: Relapse following discontinuation of lithium maintenance therapy in adolescents with bipolar I illness: a naturalistic study. Am J Psychiatry 147:457–461, 1990

Strober M, DeAntonio M, Schmidt-Lackner S, et al: Early childhood attention deficit hyperactivity disorder predicts poorer response to acute lithium therapy in adolescent mania. J Affect Disord 51:145–151, 1998

Suppes T, Chisholm KA, Dhavale D, et al: Tiagabine in treatment refractory bipolar disorder: a clinical case series. Bipolar Disord 4:283–289, 2002

Swope GS, Hoopes SP, Amy LS: An open-label study of lamotrigine in adolescents with bipolar mood disorder. Presented at the 157th annual meeting of the American Psychiatric Association. New York, May 2004

Teitelbaum M: Oxcarbazepine in bipolar disorder. J Am Acad Child Adolesc Psychiatry 40:993–994, 2001

Tillman R, Geller B, Bolhofner K, et al: Ages of onset and rates of syndromal and subsyndromal comorbid DSM-IV diagnoses in a prepubertal and early adolescent bipolar disorder phenotype. J Am Acad Child Adolesc Psychiatry 42:1486–1493, 2003

Uldall P, Bulteau C, Pedersen SA, et al: Tiagabine adjunctive therapy in children with refractory epilepsy: a single-blind dose escalating study. Epilepsy Res 42:159–168, 2000

Varanka TM, Weller RA, Weller EB, et al: Lithium treatment of manic episodes with psychotic features in prepubertal children. Am J Psychiatry 145:1557–1559, 1988

Wagner KD, Weller EB, Carlson GA, et al: An open-label trial of divalproex in children and adolescents with bipolar disorder. J Am Acad Child Adolesc Psychiatry 41:1224–1230, 2002

West SA, Keck PE Jr, McElroy SL: Open trial of valproate in the treatment of adolescent mania. J Child Adolesc Psychopharmacol 4:263–267, 1994

Williams JB: Adverse effects of thyroid hormones. Drugs Aging 11:460–469, 1997

Woolston JL: Case study: carbamazepine treatment of juvenile-onset bipolar disorder. J Am Acad Child Adolesc Psychiatry 38:335–338, 1999

Chapter 7

Special Considerations for Women With Bipolar Disorder

Natalie L. Rasgon, M.D., Ph.D.
Laurel N. Zappert, B.A.

Bipolar disorder is a cyclical disorder characterized by multiple phases of euphoria and/or dysphoria followed by intermittent periods of mood stability. Bipolar disorder carries a high rate of relapse, and half of all patients experience a second mood episode within 1 year of recovery from a previous episode (Solomon et al. 1995). More than 90% of patients who have an initial episode of mania will subsequently have one or more manic episodes. These recurring episodes have been demonstrated to have a cumulative deteriorative effect on patient functioning and recovery (American Psychiatric Association 2000; Gelenberg and Hopkins 1996). Patients with bipolar disorder frequently experience disruption in interpersonal relationships and employment and have difficulty maintaining or sustaining social support. Hospitalizations related to the disorder are common, and health care utilization costs are high, creating a significant drain on societal resources (Frye and Altshuler 1997). These factors make early identification and treatment vital to the course and prognosis of bipolar disorder.

Although the prevalence of bipolar disorder is equal between sexes, the presentation in men and women may differ, and a number of special considerations must be taken into account when treating female bipolar patients (Burt and Rasgon 2004).

Questions include:

- What are the reasons women may be more likely to develop severe forms of the illness such as rapid cycling?
- What is the relationship between the phases of reproductive life (e.g., menarche, menstrual cycle, pregnancy, and menopause) and the course of bipolar disorder?
- What are the effects of medications on neuroendocrine function in women with bipolar disorder?
- What are the effects of medication in pregnant and breastfeeding women with bipolar disorder?

This chapter reviews the evidence for special considerations in bipolar women and the data for best clinical practice in the management of these women.

Epidemiology

The prevalence of bipolar disorder has been found to be approximately 1.2% of the United States population aged 18 years and older (Regier et al. 1993). Therefore, more than 1.5 million people are affected by the disorder in the United States alone (Frye and Altshuler 1997). The age of onset for bipolar disorder is usually in the reproductive years, with the mean age of onset generally reported in the late teens to mid-20s (Goodwin and Jamison 1990). Approximately 10%–15% of adolescents with recurrent major depressive episodes will later develop bipolar I disorder (American Psychiatric Association 2000). In adolescents and young adults, mixed episodes appear to be much more likely than in older adults. It should be noted that in adolescents and young adults, a much higher prevalence rate has been reported for the entire spectrum of bipolar disorders (including bipolar disorder I, bipolar disorder II, cyclothymia, and bipolar disorder not otherwise specified), with rates ranging between 2.6% and 6.5% (Angst 1998).

Neuroendocrine Function in Bipolar Disorder

The neuroendocrine systems, which play integral roles in mood regulation, are dysfunctional in patients with affective disorders.

An anatomic study conducted by Sassi et al. (2001) using magnetic resonance imaging found that patients diagnosed with bipolar disorder had significantly smaller pituitary volumes compared with patients with unipolar depression or healthy control subjects. In neuroendocrine challenge studies, bipolar disorder is characterized by abnormalities of hypothalamic-pituitary-adrenal (HPA) function as seen primarily in a blunted response in the dexamethasone suppression test (Rush et al. 1997; Rybakowski and Twardowska 1999; Schmider et al. 1995); blunted prolactin and growth hormone responses to fenfluramine and dexamethasone (Lichtenberg et al. 1992; Thakore and Dinan 1996; Thakore et al. 1996); and blunted release of thyrotropin-stimulating hormone in response to administration of exogenous thyrotropin-releasing hormone (Rush et al. 1997). Central dysfunction of serotonergic neurotransmission may contribute to some or all of these abnormalities. Finally, a high incidence of menstrual irregularities reflecting hypothalamic-pituitary-gonadal (HPG) axis dysregulation has been observed in clinical studies of patients with bipolar disorder.

The degree to which these functional, anatomical, and clinical neuroendocrine abnormalities cause or result from mood pathology—or both—is difficult to ascertain on the basis of currently available data. The primary clinical manifestation of neuroendocrine dysfunction in bipolar disorder is likely the illness itself. Specifically, abnormalities in the neuroendocrine system with or without other central or peripheral nervous system pathologies may contribute importantly to the pathophysiological basis of bipolar disorder.

Further research is necessary before the clinical significance of neuroendocrine abnormalities in bipolar disorder is properly understood. Additionally, more research is needed to define the clinical implications of specific aspects of neuroendocrine dysfunction in bipolar disorder. Research should assess the degree to which specific hormonal responses that are blunted in bipolar disorder contribute to mood symptoms and the impact of medications that normalize specific aspects of neuroendocrine function on mood symptoms.

Sex Differences

Bipolar disorder affects similar numbers of males and females; however, research has suggested significant sex differences in symptom presentation. Whereas bipolar I disorder affects men and women in equal proportions, bipolar II and rapid-cycling subtypes are overrepresented in women (Tondo and Baldessarini 1998). Many studies have noted differences in the clinical course of bipolar disorder between the sexes, with women tending to have depressive (Angst 1978; Perugi et al. 1990) and mixed (McElroy et al. 1995; Taylor and Abrams 1981) episodes and rapid cycling (Coryell et al. 1992) more frequently than men. While depressed, women may experience atypical features more often than men (Benazzi 1999).

The etiology and course of seasonal affective disorder and rapid-cycling mood disorders suggests that reproductive hormones may contribute importantly to the course of affective illness during different menstrual cycle phases (Rubinow 1995). In addition, an increased vulnerability for mood episodes in women with bipolar disorder has been reported in relation to childbearing, the premenstrual period, and the menopausal transition (Blehar et al. 1998).

The number and type of manic episodes also appears to be related to sex. In females, the first affective episode appears more likely to be a major depressive episode, whereas the first episode in males may be more likely to be a manic episode. In women, major depressive episodes predominate, whereas in men the occurrences of manic episodes equal or exceed the number of major depressive episodes (American Psychiatric Association 2000). Rapid cycling (Robb et al. 1998) and mixed mania (Arnold et al. 2000; Robb et al. 1998; Tondo and Baldessarini 1998) also occur with much greater frequency in women, and both are associated with a poorer prognosis (Keller et al. 1986). A recent study by Rasgon et al. (2002) determined that women not only were more likely to be depressed but also were more likely than men to have cyclical changes in mood. Women with bipolar disorder are also more likely to experience later onset of mania, impaired physical health, and pain disorders (Robb et al. 1998). In addition, compared with bipolar men (49.1%), fewer bipolar women (29.1%) have a lifetime history of alcoholism (Frye et al. 2003). However, bipolar women had a much greater likelihood of alcoholism compared with the general female population, than did bipolar men when compared with the general male population (Frye et al. 2003).

Differences in treatment response may be attributed to the differences in the clinical presentation between women and men. Although Viguera et al. (2000b) found no sex differences in response to lithium in their review of 17 studies, Freeman and McElroy (1999) noted that mixed states (which respond more poorly to lithium) occurred more frequently in women. Women may also be at higher risk for receiving antidepressant treatment, because depressive symptoms are the even more pervasive in women than in men with bipolar disorder. It is therefore plausible that some of the risk for rapid cycling in women may reflect greater exposure to the mood-destabilizing effects of antidepressants (Tondo and Baldessarini 1998). Leibenluft (1997) suggested that women may also be at higher risk of antidepressant-induced hypomania or mania than men. It is therefore of particular importance to optimize use of mood stabilizers and only use antidepressants adjunctively and with substantial caution, because antidepressants may be a factor in the development of mania and cycle acceleration in women (Leibenluft 1997).

Whereas lithium has only modest efficacy (Dunner and Fieve 1974), early reports suggested that valproate, carbamazepine, and clozapine were useful for patients with rapid-cycling bipolar disorder (Leibenluft 1997). As described in Chapter 5, later studies suggest that rapid cycling may be resistant to diverse treatments. Importantly, valproate appears less effective in treating depressive symptoms (which predominate in rapid-cycling bipolar disorder) than in treating mania. Although both valproate and carbamazepine were cited in early studies as being effective in treating rapid cycling, later work suggested that these medications often require adjunctive agents, including lithium and antidepressants (Leibenluft 1997). One recent study found that even the combination of lithium and valproate yielded only modest benefit in rapid cycling (Calabrese 2003) (see Chapter 3).

Reports have demonstrated lamotrigine's efficacy in bipolar

depression (Calabrese et al. 1999), and possibly in rapid cycling (Calabrese et al. 2000). Despite encouraging early open reports, later controlled trials suggested that gabapentin and topiramate are not effective as primary therapies in bipolar disorder but may be useful adjuncts for mood or comorbid symptoms.

Although systematic clinical trials that could clarify this issue are lacking, some anticonvulsant mood stabilizers may be more appropriate for use in female patients because they are more effective in treating depressive or mixed symptoms and rapid cycling without increasing the risk of escalation to hypomania or mania. These and other sex differences warrant discussion of special considerations in the treatment of women with bipolar disorder.

Relationship Between Mood and Menstrual Cycle

The premenstrual period may be associated with worsening of ongoing major depressive, manic, mixed, or hypomanic episodes (American Psychiatric Association 2000); however, the exact nature of this relationship has yet to be elucidated. In reproductive-age women with affective disorders, the premenstrual and menstrual phases of the cycle have been associated with increased rates of suicide attempts, increased severity of suicidal intent, and increased rates of psychiatric hospitalization (Diamond et al. 1976). Premenstrual worsening of mood in women with bipolar disorder may be related to premenstrual dysphoric disorder (PMDD), because a significant overlap has been reported between the clinical manifestations of affective disorders and PMDD (Schmidt et al. 1997). In some women with prospectively documented PMDD, premenstrual dysphoria and other affective changes are followed by rapid postmenstrual changes to euthymia or euphoria, similar to mood state switches observed in bipolar disorder (Rubinow et al. 1988). PMDD and bipolar disorder may coexist, or a long-standing PMDD may evolve into bipolar disorder (Schmidt et al. 1991) by "spreading" into previously quiescent phases of the menstrual cycle. Both disorders have similar characteristic cyclic mood swings and many putative neurochemical similarities.

Cyclic changes in endorphin and catecholamine levels occur

in both PMDD and bipolar disorder (Price and DiMarzio 1986). The principal metabolite of central nervous system norepinephrine, 3-methoxy-4-hydroxyphenylglycol (MHPG), is elevated during the luteal phase of the menstrual cycle and rapidly declines 2 days prior to menses (DeLeon et al. 1978). Similarly, MHPG is elevated during manic states of bipolar disorder and may be decreased during depressive episodes (Goodwin and Jamison 1990). In addition, serotonin has been implicated in both disorders (Price and DiMarzio 1986), because L-tryptophan (the serotonin precursor) and pyridoxine (a cofactor in the decarboxylative synthesis of serotonin) have been used in successful treatment of both PMDD (Abraham and Hargrove 1980; Price et al. 1985) and affective disorders (Adams et al. 1973; VanPraag 1981).

Results from analyses of relationships between mood and the menstrual cycle in women with bipolar disorder are variable. Although early analyses suggested a relationship between mood and menstrual cycles (Endo et al. 1978), other reports have not found a specific connection between menstrual cycle and bipolar disorder (Leibenluft et al. 1999; Wehr et al. 1988). Prospective studies can provide the most accurate ratings of menstrual cycle–related mood changes, yet few studies have been published that use such methodology. One case report of a woman with schizoaffective disorder followed longitudinally for 11 years illustrated a predictable occurrence of manic episodes during the paramenstrual or follicular phase of her menstrual cycle (Bauer et al. 2001). Another case report used ChronoRecord software to prospectively document improvement in chronic monthly cycling with follicular phase depression and luteal phase hypomania when venlafaxine was discontinued and lamotrigine was added to valproate (Becker et al., in press).

In a recent pilot study (Rasgon et al. 2003), we investigated the influence of the menstrual cycle on mood in women with bipolar disorder who were taking medication but were not selected for menstrual abnormalities. We found that the majority of reproductive-aged women with bipolar illness taking medication (65%) reported significant mood changes across the menstrual cycle. However, there was no clear pattern to the direction of mood changes across the menstrual cycle. These findings replicated the earlier findings of Leibenluft et al. (1999), who examined mood in patients with rapid-cycling bipolar disorder. Leibenluft and colleagues had found that 11 of 25 women reported significant mood changes in relation to menstrual cycle, but with no consistent pattern of change. This finding is in agreement with several (Blehar et al. 1998; Leibenluft et al. 1999; Printz et al. 2001; Wehr 1990), but not all (Schmidt et al. 1990), reports.

We also found that 59% of women treated for bipolar disorder had long (>29 days) menstrual cycles with 18% displaying oligomenorrhea. This finding is consistent with a previous report that menstrual abnormalities are common in women with bipolar disorder who are receiving mood stabilizers (Rasgon et al. 2003). Although it is possible that long menstrual cycles resulted from the pharmacological treatment of bipolar disorder, the previous observation of menstrual abnormalities preceding the onset of bipolar symptoms and current observation of long menstrual cycles in the presence of oral contraceptive use suggest that there may be a underlying vulnerability to long or abnormal menstrual cycles in women with bipolar disorder (Rasgon et al. 2003).

Mood changes across the menstrual cycle, and the effects of long menstrual cycles on the course of bipolar disorder, warrant investigation not only because of their theoretical implications but also because of their clinical consequences. Recent reports suggest increased appreciation of the significance of menstrual abnormalities in reproductive-aged women, because menstrual abnormalities may be a marker of associated metabolic abnormalities, including a predictor of increased risk for non–insulin dependent diabetes (Solomon et al. 2001).

Treatment Considerations

Pharmacotherapy, including the use of mood stabilizers (lithium, valproate, and carbamazepine) and atypical antipsychotics, has been the foundation of treatment for patients with bipolar disorder. Lithium and some anticonvulsants (valproate, carbamazepine, lamotrigine) have demonstrated acute and/or prophylactic efficacy in bipolar disorder. It should be noted that these medications have been shown to alter endocrine function

(Goodwin and Jamison 1990), and treatment decisions must therefore include careful consideration of the interactions between mood stabilizers and endocrine function.

Weight Gain

Antipsychotic and antidepressant use in patients has been found to be related to increased rates of impaired glucose tolerance and diabetes (Muller-Oerlinghausen et al. 1978; Paykel et al. 1973). A common adverse effect of pharmacotherapy for bipolar disorder is weight gain, with a predominant increase in central adiposity (Vestergaard et al. 1988). It has been clearly established that excess body fat with this distribution is associated with the "metabolic syndrome" (Saltar et al. 1998) as well as an increased risk for ischemic heart disease, type 2 diabetes mellitus, gall bladder disease, osteoarthritis, and some cancers (Pi–Sunyer 1991). In addition, weight gain may prompt patients to discontinue treatment, with consequent reductions in treatment efficacy and social functioning (Gitlin et al. 1989).

The study of obesity prevalence in bipolar disorder is limited; however, uncontrolled data are available for schizophrenia patients. In uncontrolled studies of patients with schizophrenia treated with lithium, the prevalence of obesity has been reported to be two to five times higher than in the general population (Chen and Silverstone 1990; Muller-Oerlinghausen et al. 1978). Similarly, a two- to fourfold increase in obesity has been reported among those treated with antipsychotics (Gopalaswarny and Morgan 1985; Silverstone et al. 1988). Even higher rates have been observed in female patients. One study found that 59% of female epilepsy patients receiving valproate were obese (Isojarvi et al. 1996). A study conducted by Elmslie et al. (2000) evaluated the prevalence of overweight and obesity in patients with bipolar disorder and replicated the results found in previously mentioned studies. They found that female bipolar patients treated with lithium experienced more weight gain than men and that excess weight and obesity are more frequent in women treated with antipsychotics. Emerging data suggest that obese compared with nonobese bipolar disorder patients have poorer outcome (Fagiolini et al. 2003).

Strategies should be developed to limit weight gain in bipolar patients, especially women and those who require antipsychotic medication. The Stanley Foundation Bipolar Network is evaluating the effectiveness of two medications with anorectic properties, sibutramine (Meridia) and topiramate (Topamax), in the treatment of psychotropic drug-associated weight gain in patients with bipolar disorder. Topiramate treatment of patients with epilepsy and bipolar disorder has been associated with weight loss. In clinical epilepsy trials, among topiramate-treated patients with seizures, mean decreases in weight from baseline to endpoint ranged from 1.3 kg (1.7% decline) in the lowest dosage group (<200 mg/day) to 6.1 kg (7.2%) in the highest dosage group (>800 mg/day). In addition, patients who weighed the most (>100 kg) before topiramate treatment displayed the greatest weight loss (average loss of 8.6 kg compared with 1.3 kg for patients weighing <60 kg). Women also tended to experience more weight loss compared with men of comparable baseline weight. Recent data from patients with bipolar disorder who gained substantial amounts of weight associated with psychotropic treatment regimens (e.g., lithium, valproate, conventional and atypical antipsychotics, some antidepressants) also suggest that topiramate may be effective in reducing weight gain in patients with bipolar illness as well as in patients with epilepsy (McElroy 1998). For example, 18 patients with bipolar disorder with a mean baseline weight of 241 lb displayed a mean weight loss of 14 lb over a 5-month interval when treated with topiramate (mean dosage 343 mg/day). In all cases, topiramate was added to ongoing treatment regimens. In general, the addition of topiramate was well tolerated. Sibutramine has not yet been systematically studied in the treatment of weight gain associated with psychotropic drugs, and only open label, uncontrolled pilot data are available regarding the efficacy and safety of sibutramine for this syndrome (McElroy 1998). Possible antidepressant properties have been attributed to sibutramine because of its reuptake inhibition of serotonin, norepinephrine, and dopamine (Weintraub et al. 1991). Controlled data suggest zonisamide yields weight loss in obesity (Gadde et al. 2003), and preliminary open data suggest this agent may also permit weight loss in obese bipolar disorder patients (McElroy 2003; Yang et al. 2003).

Treatment Across the Menstrual Cycle

In women, treatment efficacy may vary across the menstrual cycle. Two well-documented cases indicated that serum lithium levels vary in relation to the menstrual cycle in some women with catamenial bipolar symptoms (Conrad and Hamilton 1986). In bipolar women followed longitudinally, serum lithium levels were increased during depression and decreased during mania (Kukopulos and Reginaldi 1978), whereas in asymptomatic women, lithium levels remained constant over the menstrual cycle (Chamberlain et al. 1990). The mechanism by which bipolar disorder may be entrained to the menstrual cycle remains unknown.

Medication Effects on Reproductive Function

Mood stabilizers, anticonvulsants, and some antipsychotics may influence serum levels of reproductive hormones and consequently impact reproductive function. In women, the investigation of the effects of these medications on reproductive endocrine function is especially crucial. Although atypical antipsychotics generally have modest effects on prolactin, risperidone and typical antipsychotics can yield clinically significant prolactin elevation, resulting in galactorrhea, menstrual irregularities, and problems with sexual desire and function. Serotonin reuptake inhibitors, although useful for PMDD and depressive symptoms, may not only destabilize mood but also impair sexual desire and function.

There are large gaps in our knowledge of the effects of anticonvulsants on the reproductive endocrine function of women with bipolar disorder. Only one study has been published to date that specifically addresses medication effects on reproductive endocrine function in women with bipolar disorder (Rasgon et al. 2000). However, several reports have been published that have addressed this topic in women with epilepsy. Some studies in the 1990s suggested an association between anticonvulsants used in treating epilepsy and reproductive abnormalities in women, ranging from menstrual dysfunction to polycystic ovary syndrome (PCOS). However, no consensus has been reached as to whether manifestation of menstrual abnormalities in women with epilepsy is related to anticonvulsants, epilepsy, or an interaction between anticonvulsants and epilepsy.

Polycystic Ovary Syndrome

PCOS is the most common endocrine disorder in women of reproductive age (Franks 1995). PCOS is characterized by androgen hypersecretion (hyperandrogenism), insulin resistance, and chronic anovulation in the absence of specific underlying diseases of the adrenal or pituitary glands (Franks 1995). In spite of its name, PCOS does not by definition require the presence of polycystic ovaries, although these are very common. Clinical manifestations include hirsutism, seborrhea, acne, alopecia, menstrual irregularities, obesity, and infertility (Dunaif et al. 1989).

Anovulation resulting from PCOS may manifest clinically as amenorrhea or irregular menses and ultimately may result in infertility. Other endocrine abnormalities have been associated with PCOS, including fasting and glucose stimulated hyperinsulinemia, peripheral insulin resistance, and chronically elevated plasma-free estrogen and testosterone levels (Franks 1995). In addition, approximately 50% of women with PCOS are obese (Dunaif et al. 1988; Pasquali and Cassimirri 1993), which may contribute to insulin resistance and other symptoms of PCOS (Dunaif and Thomas 2001).

The increased serum testosterone levels in PCOS can be the result of androgen overproduction by the adrenal glands and ovaries (Gonzalez 1997). Hyperandrogenism can lead to insulin resistance and hyperinsulinemia, and vice versa (Dunaif et al. 1989). Hyperinsulinemia plays a significant role in the development of PCOS, because insulin promotes androgen production by ovarian thecal cells (Yen 1991). Obesity alone increases the risk of insulin resistance, although insulin resistance can occur in the absence of obesity (Chang et al. 1983; Dunaif et al. 1989). The use of oral contraceptives can interrupt the cycle of hyperandrogenism and insulin resistance by modulating the HPG regulatory system (Yen 1991).

The fundamental defect in the PCOS is unclear, but theories implicate dysfunction of the HPG and HPA axes and related neurochemical systems. One theory suggests that exaggerated maturation of the adrenal system (adrenarche) in obese girls leads to insulin resistance (Yen 1991). Other theories propose insulin resistance as a critical pathogenic mechanism, which is supported by the finding that women with PCOS show greater prevalence of glucose intolerance and frank type 2 diabetes mellitus (Pierpoint et al. 1998).

Polycystic Ovary Syndrome in Women With Epilepsy

Regardless of treatment, women with epilepsy, compared with healthy women, demonstrate an increased prevalence of PCOS (Herzog et al. 1984). Initial studies of relationships between epilepsy and PCOS were conducted by Isojarvi et al. (1993, 1996). Results of these studies, however, are complicated by pharmacotherapy, because anticonvulsants (such as valproate and carbamazepine) often used to treat epilepsy may change the serum concentrations of sex hormones (Isojarvi et al. 1991). Anticonvulsants have been reported to change the metabolism of reproductive hormones, including estrogen, progesterone, and testosterone, with resultant alteration of circulating blood levels of these hormones and secondary effects on the feedback loop of the HPG axis (Mattson and Cramer 1985). Carbamazepine can induce hepatic enzymes including the cytochrome P450 3A4 isoform, causing not only autoinduction of its own metabolism but also an increased metabolism of ovarian steroids, including estrogen, progesterone, and testosterone. Furthermore, carbamazepine increases levels of sex hormone–binding globulin and secondarily lowers free testosterone levels, resulting in a modest elevation of serum gonadotropins, (i.e., follicle-stimulating and luteinizing hormones) (Margraf and Dreifuss 1981; Mattson and Cramer 1985). Despite these alterations in serum sex hormone concentrations, menstrual cycles appear to remain ovulatory in women treated with carbamazepine (Isojarvi et al. 1993). Finally, endocrine and metabolic consequences of PCOS may include coronary heart disease, hypertension, diabetes, and cancer. The importance of these consequences and their clinical implications has stimulated further investigation of the effect of anticonvulsants on female reproductive function.

Polycystic Ovary Syndrome in Women With Bipolar Disorder

An unequivocal association between treatment of bipolar disorder and reproductive endocrine function has not been established (O'Donovan et al. 2002). To date, information regarding the risk of developing PCOS with valproate use in the bipolar female population is still emerging (Burt and Rasgon 2004). Several case reports describe PCOS-like changes in women with various psychiatric illnesses (Ghazuidin 1989; Petho et al. 1982). A study by Matsunaga and Sarai (1993) evaluated the HPG axes of 12 women with bipolar or psychotic symptoms that fluctuated in association with their menstrual cycles. Several hormonal features were observed, including elevated basal luteinizing hormone ($n=8$; 67%) and decreased basal follicle-stimulating hormone ($n=6$; 50%). Polycystic ovaries were observed by ultrasonography in 8 (67%) of the 12 patients. The authors suggested that a relationship may exist between the psychiatric disorders and PCOS-associated hormonal abnormalities in these cases. Their findings however, may be confounded by the use of antipsychotic medications at the time of the investigation, which are known to alter the HPG function via hyperprolactinemia, and by the use of oral contraceptive by one patient.

In a study by Rasgon et al. (2003), mood, menstrual, psychiatric, and life event data were collected prospectively for 17 women with bipolar disorder for 3 consecutive months. All women received medications for bipolar disorder; in addition, 35% of the women received oral contraceptives. The investigators reported that 59% of women treated for bipolar disorder had long (>29 days) menstrual cycle length, with 18% displaying oligomenorrhea. These results are consistent with an earlier report indicating that menstrual abnormalities are common in women with bipolar disorder (Rasgon et al. 2000). Although it is possible

that the abnormal menstrual cycles are a result of pharmacotherapy in these studies, the observations that menstrual abnormalities precede the onset of bipolar symptoms and that
simultaneous oral contraceptive use is associated with long menstrual cycles suggest that women with bipolar disorder may have
an underlying predisposition to long or abnormal menstrual cycles (Matsunaga and Sarai 1993; Rasgon et al. 2003).

Emerging data are beginning to reveal the prevalence of
PCOS in women with bipolar disorder who are receiving mood
stabilizers. Preliminary data from the Systematic Treatment Enhancement Program for Bipolar Disorder study suggest that in
adult females, valproate use may carry a modest risk of PCOS, as
9 of 86 women (10.5%) taking valproate developed PCOS. Altshuler et al. (2004) recently examined serum reproductive
hormone levels in 72 women with bipolar disorder taking mood-
stabilizing medications to determine whether receiving
valproate impaired reproductive or metabolic hormone levels.
Across the entire sample, mean levels of homeostasis model assessment, luteinizing hormone and follicle stimulating hormone
ratios, and prolactin were increased and mean levels of estrogen
were decreased. Women given valproate compared with those
not given valproate had similar mean free and total testosterone
levels. Additionally, three women in the group receiving valproate (6%) met criteria for PCOS, a proportion comparable with
population rates and not significantly different from the group
not receiving valproate. Of those women who did not have menstrual abnormalities prior to treatment, no significant differences
emerged between groups as assessed by either mean hormone
levels or the proportion of women outside the clinically normal
range. Further studies are needed in this area, including assessments of the risk of PCOS with valproate use in adolescent females.

Oral Contraceptives and Bipolar Disorder

A major concern for women of childbearing age is the efficacy of
oral contraceptives, and this should be considered when initiating therapy for bipolar disorder because some medications may

alter the efficacy of oral contraceptives (Burt and Rasgon 2004). Mood stabilizers such as carbamazepine, and to a lesser extent oxcarbazepine and topiramate (for the latter, especially above 200 mg/day), may affect the metabolism of oral contraceptives presumably by inducing hepatic cytochrome P450 activity and thus decreasing levels of oral contraceptives (Crawford 2002).

In addition, the efficacy of other medications may likewise be altered by oral contraceptive. Sabers et al. (2001) presented a case series of seven women with epilepsy who received oral contraceptives while being treated with lamotrigine to determine the contraceptives' effect on lamotrigine plasma levels. Overall, oral contraceptives reduced lamotrigine plasma levels by 41%–64%, with a mean decrease in plasma lamotrigine levels of 49%. The authors concluded that women with epilepsy who are treated with both lamotrigine and oral contraceptive should have their lamotrigine plasma levels monitored closely and their lamotrigine dosage adjusted as necessary. No drug interactions with oral contraceptives have been reported to date with valproate, lithium, gabapentin, or the atypical antipsychotics (Physicians' Desk Reference 2004).

The potential mood-stabilizing effects of oral contraceptives in women should be noted. In the previously mentioned study of mood changes across the menstrual cycle (Rasgon et al. 2003); women taking oral contraceptives did not have significant mood changes, whereas those not taking oral contraceptives did have significant mood changes. This finding is consistent with several studies that have reported the mood-stabilizing effects of exogenous gonadal steroids in women with treatment-resistant bipolar disorder (Chouinard et al. 1987; Hatotani et al. 1983; Price and Giannini 1985). Similar effects in women with PCOS have been observed, because oral contraceptive treatment has been associated with decreased rates of depression (Pearlstein and Steiner 2000). Our findings suggest that in women with bipolar disorder, oral contraceptives may have mood-stabilizing effects premenstrually (Rasgon et al. 2003). Indeed oral contraceptives are effective in attenuating symptoms of PCOS itself. Women with premenstrual syndrome represent another population for whom oral contraceptives may ameliorate perimenstrual mood changes (Patten and

Lamarre 1992). However, some women with bipolar disorder report that oral contraceptives exacerbate mood problems.

In healthy women, exogenous gonadal steroids, such as those used for oral contraception or hormonal replacement, can affect mood negatively (Price and DiMarzio 1986). Thus, some bipolar women, as well as some women with PCOS and premenstrual syndrome, may represent subpopulations for whom oral contraceptives may have mood-stabilizing effects. Taken together, these studies of the effects of oral contraceptives on those patients with endocrine and mood disorders may represent a link between reproductive endocrine dysfunction and affective illness. Because the effects of oral contraceptives are heterogeneous, clinicians need to ascertain whether oral contraceptives affect mood positively, negatively, or not at all in individual patients.

Treatment During Pregnancy

In pregnant bipolar patients, the potential for the development of adverse fetal or neonatal adverse effects should be considered when assessing the use of medications (Burt and Rasgon 2004). Potential side effects include intrauterine death, perinatal toxicity, teratogenicity, growth retardation, and neurobehavioral toxicity (Holmes et al. 2001). Other considerations include special treatment issues associated with pregnancy (e.g., the need for dosage adjustments) and risk of recurrence and exacerbation of mood episodes. Substantial risk for relapse has been found to exist during the pregnancy period following discontinuation of mood-stabilizing medication (Viguera et al. 2002a). Viguera et al. (2000a) found similar rates of recurrence during the first 40 weeks after lithium discontinuation for pregnant (52%) and nonpregnant women (58%); however, relapse rates had been much lower for both groups in the year before lithium was discontinued (21%).

As previously discussed, information remains limited regarding the risk for recurrence of bipolar disorder in pregnant women after discontinuation of lithium or other mood stabilizers. Teratogenic effects of lithium (Epstein's anomaly in 0.1%; Cohen et al. 1994), valproate (neural tube defects in 1%–2%;

Omtzigt et al. 1992), and carbamazepine (spina bifida in 3%, craniofacial defects in 11%, fingernail hypoplasia in 26%, and developmental delay in 20%) have been described (Jones et al. 1989; Rosa 1991). Recent data suggest that rates of malformation with divalproex could be higher compared to rates with lamotrigine or compared to rates with no anticonvulsant exposure (Alsdorf et al. 2004; Cunnington 2004; Vajda et al. 2004). Less is known regarding teratogenicity of most atypical antipsychotics and other anticonvulsants, many of which have emerged more recently. A preliminary study demonstrated no increased risk of teratogenicity in 23 cases during which olanzapine was used antenatally (Goldstein et al. 2000). Recent data suggest that rates of malformations with lamotrigine are similar to those encountered in the general population, and lower than those with valproate (Cunnington 2004).

Teratogenic effects in pregnancy have not been demonstrated with use of verapamil. In a preliminary naturalistic study of 37 bipolar women, Wisner et al. (2002) found that verapamil was effective for acute treatment of mania and for prevention of bipolar recurrence when used as a maintenance medication. However, more adequately powered controlled studies are necessary to ascertain the efficacy of verapamil before it can be considered effective (Leibenluft 2000).

Although limited data suggest that lithium discontinuation during pregnancy carries similar relapse rates compared with other times, further studies are needed to assess discontinuation of medication and resulting acute psychiatric illness on fetal development (Viguera et al. 2002a). However, the following recommendations are helpful if the pregnant patient is to be treated with mood stabilizers:

- Pharmacotherapy during pregnancy should be avoided if clinically possible (Iqbal et al. 2001), especially during the first trimester. This, however, may not be possible for bipolar women who have historically demonstrated rapid relapse upon discontinuation of mood stabilizers. Discontinuation of medications in women with histories of suicidal depression or psychotic manias should be approached with particular caution.

- At least 3 months before pregnancy, prenatal counseling should be instituted and patients should be suitably educated about the known possible risks of taking medications during pregnancy, the genetic risk of transmission of bipolar disorder to offspring, and the risks to themselves and their unborn children of antenatal bipolar decompensation (Iqbal et al. 2001).
- It is important to use minimal effective dosages if psychotropics are used during pregnancy. Partial treatment carries the risks of both teratogenesis and maternal psychiatric decompensation (Llewellyn et al. 1998).
- Dosing changes related to hemodynamic changes, reduced absorption, liver metabolism changes, and decreased protein binding may be required during pregnancy. It is not uncommon for dosage requirements to rise, in part due to the increased extracellular fluid volume during pregnancy. Following delivery, pre-pregnancy doses should be reinstated unless there is acute postpartum destabilization.
- During pregnancy, monotherapy is preferred, and the minimum dosage of medication that sustains psychiatric stability should be prescribed (Iqbal et al. 2001).
- Folate supplementation 3 months before conception and continuing into the first trimester of pregnancy may reduce the risk of neural tube defects (Iqbal et al. 2001). Although daily folate supplementation of 0.4 mg is recommended for all women of childbearing age to prevent spina bifida and other neural tube defects, dosages of 4 mg/day are recommended for high-risk women who have previously delivered infants with neural tube defects. Although there are no formal guidelines for folic acid supplementation in women on valproate and carbamazepine, these women are at increased risk for having babies with neural tube defects. Therefore bipolar women on these medications should consult their treating physicians regarding whether they require a 4 mg/day supplement of folate while actively attempting pregnancy and during the first 3 months of pregnancy (American Academy of Pediatrics Committee on Drugs 2000).
- Psychotherapy may be a useful adjunctive treatment. In a recent uncontrolled small study of 13 pregnant depressed

women utilizing a modified version of interpersonal psychotherapy, all subjects appeared to respond with full remission of depressive symptoms (Spinelli 1997). Although interpersonal psychotherapy has been endorsed as a treatment for major depression with postpartum onset (O'Hara et al. 2000), there are no studies investigating the efficacy of psychotherapy in the management of bipolar disorder during pregnancy.

- An important aspect of therapy in bipolar women is to encourage the patient to seek support from family and friends for infant care, to maximize sleep, and to minimize other responsibilities. Support from the partner has been of significant benefit for women experiencing postpartum depression (Rapkin et al. 2002).
- Although electroconvulsive therapy is not a standard first-line treatment for bipolar disorder, it may be an important alternative to medication during pregnancy, especially in cases of suicidal or homicidal ideation (infanticide) or psychotic decompensation. To date, there has been no indication of teratogenesis associated with electroconvulsive therapy (Llewellyn et al. 1998), and the treatment is relatively safe during pregnancy if special precautions are taken to reduce potential risks (Miller 1994).
- In women who have psychotic decompensation during the postpartum period, treatment should be aggressive because of the risk to both mother and infant. Early treatment allows the mother to recover and proceed with mother–infant attachment. Because of the particular danger of infanticide, contact between a psychotic mother and infant needs to be regulated and supervised carefully. Hospitalization is often required, especially if the mother appears dangerous to herself or her infant (Rapkin et al. 2002).
- Recommended treatment for postpartum psychosis includes mood stabilizers (e.g., lithium); neuroleptics (high-potency antipsychotics like haloperidol are preferred over low-potency antipsychotics and are often required for severe psychosis); olanzapine; risperidone; quetiapine; and ECT (for those patients who do not respond to pharmacotherapy or whose symptoms threaten to escalate) (Rapkin et al. 2002).

Treatment During Breastfeeding

A risk of relapse, ranging from 20% to 82%, is associated with the postpartum period, and currently the decision about treatment for prophylaxis is generally decided on the basis of the patient's ability to avoid major mood episodes without medication (Viguera et al. 2002b). Studies examining the effectiveness of lithium to attenuate high postpartum risk for recurrence of bipolar disorder have found lithium treatment resulted in a two- to five-fold decrease in postpartum recurrences of bipolar disorder. Specifically, among subjects who remained stable over the first 40 weeks after lithium discontinuation, postpartum recurrences were 2.9 times more frequent than recurrences in nonpregnant women during weeks 41–64 (70% versus 24%) (Viguera et al. 2000a). For bipolar patients who choose to breastfeed, continuing antenatal psychotropic treatment into the postpartum and/or commencing prophylaxis after delivery may also pose very real problems. Many of the medications currently used to treat bipolar disorder lack sufficient data regarding use during breastfeeding. Although there are many advantages for maternal-infant bonding and infant health, breastfeeding commonly entails sleep deprivation, which can undermine psychiatric stability in bipolar patients. In addition, many medications are secreted in breast milk during lactation, posing other treatment dilemmas. Llewellyn et al. (1998) recommended close monitoring of the infant and a low threshold for cessation or suspension of breastfeeding during use of medication. In addition, because breastfeeding does not always prevent conception, it is important to educate patients about birth control options (Newport et al. 2002).

Conclusions

Women, compared with men, with bipolar disorder are significantly more likely to present with depression, mixed episodes, and rapid cycling, all of which appear to be less responsive to lithium treatment. The potential higher risk among bipolar women of being treated with antidepressants and the risks of developing rapid cycling and antidepressant-induced mania and hypomania suggest that treating women entails optimal mood stabilization and considerable caution with antidepressants. Although it is an option for treatment, valproate has stronger antimanic than antidepressant effects. Other treatment alternatives for bipolar women include the newer anticonvulsant lamotrigine, as controlled studies have demonstrated the efficacy of this agent in treating depressive symptoms and rapid cycling with little evidence of manic switching. To date, it remains to be seen whether other newer anticonvulsants have utility in female bipolar patients and whether they will produce fewer side effects (on mood and neuroendocrine function) in women. Although in general newer anticonvulsants do not appear as effective as monotherapy for mania, some of these medications may emerge as useful adjuncts in female patients for mood or comorbid symptoms. Care must be taken regarding the potential of some such agents to interfere with oral contraception.

During pregnancy, lithium, valproate, and carbamazepine entail some teratogenic risk. It remains to be established whether the newer anticonvulsants or atypical antipsychotics will emerge as safe or effective in this regard. At present, of the most commonly used mood stabilizers (lithium, carbamazepine, and valproate), lithium may carry a risk of birth defects. However, if the decision is made to treat during pregnancy, it may be most prudent to treat with an agent of proven utility in an individual patient rather than another agent with less putative teratogenicity but unproven utility in that person.

For women who are breastfeeding, lithium is contraindicated, and more data are needed to evaluate the safety of valproate, carbamazepine, and newer anticonvulsants and atypical antipsychotics for exposed breastfed babies.

The influence of the menstrual cycle, pregnancy, postpartum period, and menopause on the course of bipolar illness requires investigation. Considerably more research is needed to elucidate distinctive symptom presentations and the course of bipolar disorder in female patients. Although explanations for such differences are outside of the scope of this paper, the development of treatment guidelines and of modalities better suited to the needs of the female bipolar population are needed to optimize the management of bipolar disorder in women.

References

Abraham GE, Hargrove JT: Effect of vitamin B6 on premenstrual symptomatology in women with menstrual tension syndromes: a double-blind crossover study. Infertility 3:155–161, 1980

Adams PW, Rose DP, Folkard J, et al: Effect of pyridoxine hydrochloride (vitamin B6) upon depression associated with oral contraception. Lancet 1:897–904, 1973

Alsdorf RM, Wyszynski DF, Holms LB, et al: Evidence of increased birth defects in the offspring of women exposed to valproate during pregnancy: findings from the AED pregnancy pregistry. Birth Defects Res: Clin Mol Ter 70:245, 2004

Altshuler LL, Rasgon NL, Elman S, et al: Reproductive endocrine function in women treated for bipolar disorder: reproductive hormone levels. Presented at the 157th annual meeting of the American Psychiatric Association, New York, May 2004

American Academy of Pediatrics Committee on Drugs: Use of psychoactive medication during pregnancy and possible effects on the fetus and newborn: Committee on Drugs, American Academy of Pediatrics. Pediatrics 105:880–887, 2000

American Psychiatric Association: Diagnostic and Statistical Manual of Mental Disorders, 4th Edition, Text Revision. Washington, DC, American Psychiatric Association, 2000

Angst J: The course of affective disorders, II: typology of bipolar manic-depressive illness. Arch Psychiatr Nervenkr 226:65–73, 1978

Angst J: The emerging epidemiology of hypomania and bipolar II disorder. J Affect Disord 50:143–151, 1998

Arnold LM, McElroy SL, Keck PE Jr: The role of gender in mixed mania. Compr Psychiatry 41:83–87, 2000

Bauer M, Gyulai L, Glenn T, et al: A new clinical and research tool for bipolar disorder: ChronoRecord software for daily self-reporting of mood, sleep and medication. Bipolar Disord 3 (suppl 1):26, 2001

Becker OV, Rasgon NL, Marsh WK, et al: Lamotrigine therapy in treatment-resistant menstrually-related rapid cycling bipolar disorder: a case report. Bipolar Disord 6:435–439, 2004

Benazzi F: Gender differences in bipolar II and unipolar depressed outpatients: a 557-case study. Ann Clin Psychiatry 11:55–59, 1999

Blehar MC, Depaulo JR, Gershon ES, et al: Women with bipolar disorder: findings from the NIMH genetics initiative sample. Psychopharmacol Bull 34:239–243, 1998

Burt VK, Rasgon N: Special considerations in treating bipolar disorder in women. Bipolar Disord 6:2–13, 2004

Calabrese JR: Combination treatments: what to use and when. Presented at the 156th annual meeting of the American Psychiatric Association, San Francisco, CA, May 2003

Calabrese JR, Bowden CL, Sachs GS, et al: A double-blind placebo-controlled study of lamotrigine monotherapy in outpatients with bipolar I depression: Lamictal 602 Study Group. J Clin Psychiatry 60:79–88, 1999

Calabrese JR, Suppes T, Bowden CL, et al: A double-blind, placebo-controlled, prophylaxis study of lamotrigine in rapid-cycling bipolar disorder: Lamictal 614 Study Group. J Clin Psychiatry 61:841–850, 2000

Chamberlain S, Hahn, PM, Casson P, et al: Effect of menstrual cycle phase and oral contraceptive use on serum lithium levels after a loading dose of lithium in normal women. Am J Psychiatry 147:907–909, 1990

Chang RJ, Nakamura RM, Judd HL, et al: Insulin resistance in nonobese patients with polycystic ovarian disease. J Clin Endocrinol Metab 57:356–359, 1983

Chen Y, Silverstone T: Lithium and weight gain. Int Clin Psychopharmacol 5:217–225, 1990

Chouinard G, Steinberg S, Steiner W: Estrogen-progesterone combination: another mood stabilizer? (letter). Am J Psychiatry 144:826, 1987

Cohen LS, Friedman JM, Jefferson JW, et al: A reevaluation of risk of in utero exposure to lithium. JAMA 271:146–150, 1994

Conrad CD, Hamilton JA: Recurrent premenstrual decline in serum lithium concentration: clinical correlates and treatment implications. J Am Acad Child Psychiatry 25:852–853, 1986

Coryell W, Endicott J, Keller M: Rapidly cycling affective disorder: demographics, diagnosis, family history, and course. Arch Gen Psychiatry 49:126–131, 1992

Crawford P: Interactions between antiepileptic drugs and hormonal contraception. CNS Drugs 16:263–272, 2002

Cunnington MC: The International Lamotrigine Pregnancy Registry update for the epilepsy foundation. Epilepsia 45(11):1468, 2004

DeLeon Jones FA, Steinberg J, DeVirmejian H, et al: MHPG excretion during the menstrual cycle of women. Commun Psychopharmacol 2:267–274, 1978

Diamond SB, Rubinstein AA, Dunner DL, et al: Menstrual problems in women with affective illness. Compr Psychiatry 17:541–548, 1976

Dunaif A, Thomas A: Current concepts in the polycystic ovary syndrome. Annu Rev Med 52:401–419, 2001

Dunaif A, Mandeli J, Fluhr H, et al: The impact of obesity and chronic hyperinsulemia on gonadotropin release and gonadal steroid secretion in the polycystic ovary syndrome. J Clin Endocr Metab 66:131–139, 1988

Dunaif A, Segal KR, Futterweit W, et al: Profound peripheral insulin resistance, independent of obesity, in polycystic ovary syndrome. Diabetes 38:1165–1174, 1989

Dunner DL, Fieve RR: Clinical factors in lithium carbonate prophylaxis failure. Arch Gen Psychiatry 30:229–233, 1974

Elmslie JL, Silverstone TJ, Mann JI, et al: Prevalence of overweight and obesity in bipolar patients. J Clin Psychiatry 61:171–184, 2000

Endo M, Daiguji M, Asano Y, et al : Periodic psychosis recurring in association with menstrual cycle. J Clin Psychiatry 39:456–466, 1978

Fagiolini A, Kupfer DJ, Houck PR, et al: Obesity as a correlate of outcome in patients with bipolar I disorder. Am J Psychiatry 160:112–117, 2003

Franks S: Polycystic ovary syndrome. N Engl J Med 333:853–861, 1995

Freeman MP, McElroy SL: Clinical picture and etiologic models of mixed states. Psychiatr Clin North Am 22:535–546, vii, 1999

Frye MA, Altshuler LL: Selection of initial treatment for bipolar disorder, manic phase. Mod Probl Pharmacopsychiatry 25:88–113, 1997

Frye MA, Altshuler LL, McElroy SL, et al: Gender differences in prevalence, risk, and clinical correlates of alcoholism comorbidity in bipolar disorder. Am J Psychiatry 160:883–889, 2003

Gadde KM, Franciscy DM, Wagner HR 2nd, et al: Zonisamide for weight loss in obese adults: a randomized controlled trial. JAMA 289:1820–1825, 2003

Gelenberg AJ, Hopkins HS: Antipsychotics in bipolar disorder. J Clin Psychiatry 57 (suppl 9):49–52, 1996

Ghazuidin M: Polycystic ovary disease, manic depressive illness and mental retardation. J Ment Defic Res 33:335–338, 1989

Gitlin MJ, Cochran SD, Jamison KR: Maintenance lithium treatment: side effects and compliance. J Clin Psychiatry 50:127–131, 1989

Goldstein DJ, Corbin LA, Fung MC: Olanzapine-exposed pregnancies and lactation: early experience. J Clin Psychopharmacol 20:399–403, 2000

Gonzalez F: Adrenal involvement in polycystic ovary syndrome. Semin Reprod Endocrinol 15:137–157, 1997

Goodwin FK, Jamison KR: Biomedical and pharmacological studies, in Manic-Depressive Illness. New York, Oxford University Press, 1990, pp 416–502

Gopalaswarny AK, Morgan R: Too many chronically mentally disabled patients are too fat. Acta Psychiatry Scand 72:254–258, 1985

Hatotani N, Kitayama I, Inoue K, et al: Psychoendocrine studies of recurrent psychoses, in Neurobiology of Periodic Psychoses. Edited by Hatotani N, Nomura J. Tokyo, Japan, Igaku-Shoin, 1983, pp 77–92

Herzog AG, Seibel MM, Schomer DL, et al: Temporal lobe epilepsy: an extrahypothalamic pathogenesis for polycystic ovarian syndrome? Neurology 34:1389–1393, 1984

Holmes LB, Harvey EA, Coull BA, et al: The teratogenicity of anticonvulsant drugs. N Engl J Med 344:1132–1138, 2001

Iqbal MM, Gundlapalli SP, Ryan WG, et al: Effects of antimanic mood-stabilizing drugs on fetuses, neonates, and nursing infants. South Med J 94:304–322, 2001

Isojarvi JIT, Pakarinen AJ, Myllyla VV: A prospective study of serum sex hormones during carbamazepine therapy. Epilepsia 31:438–445, 1991

Isojarvi JI, Laatikainen TJ, Pakarinen AJ, et al: Polycystic ovaries and hyperandrogenism in women taking valproate for epilepsy. N Engl J Med 329:1383–1388, 1993

Isojarvi JI, Laatikainen TJ, Knip M, et al: Obesity and endocrine disorders in women taking valproate for epilepsy. Ann Neurol 39:579–584, 1996

Jones KL, Lacro RV, Johnson KA, et al: Pattern of malformations in the children of women treated with carbamazepine during pregnancy. N Engl J Med 320:1661–1666, 1989

Keller MB, Lavori PW, Coryell W, et al : Differential outcome of pure manic, mixed/cycling, and pure depressive episodes in patients with bipolar illness. JAMA 255:3138–3142, 1986

Kukopulos A, Reginaldi D: Variations of serum lithium concentrations correlated with the phases of manic-depressive psychosis. Agressologie 19:219–222, 1978

Leibenluft E: Issues in the treatment of women with bipolar illness. J Clin Psychiatry 58 (suppl 15):5–11, 1997

Leibenluft E: Women and bipolar disorder: an update. Bull Menninger Clin 64:5–17, 2000

Leibenluft E, Ashman SB, Feldman-Naim S, et al: Lack of relationship between menstrual cycle phase and mood in a sample of women with rapid cycling bipolar disorder. Biol Psychiatry 46:577–580, 1999

Lichtenberg P, Shapira B, Gillon D, et al: Hormone responses to fenflu-ramine and placebo challenge in endogenous depression. Psychiatry Res 43:137–146, 1992

Llewellyn A, Stowe ZN, Strader JR Jr: The use of lithium and manage-ment of women with bipolar disorder during pregnancy and lacta-tion. J Clin Psychiatry 59 (suppl 6):57–64, 1998

Margraf JW, Dreifuss FE: Ammenorrhea following initiation of therapy with valproic acid (abstract). Neurology 31 (suppl 159):261, 1981

Matsunaga H, Sarai M: Elevated serum LH and androgens in affective disorder related to the menstrual cycle: with reference to polycystic ovary syndrome. Jpn J Psychiatry Neurol 47:825–842, 1993

Mattson RH, Cramer JA: Epilepsy, sex hormones and antiepileptic drugs. Epilepsia 26 (suppl 1):S40–S51, 1985

McElroy SL: A pilot trial of adjunctive topiramate in the treatment of bi-polar disorder. Presented at the 21st Congress of the Collegium Inter-nationale Neuro-Psychopharmacologicum, Glasgow, Scotland, July 1998

McElroy SL: Eating disorders and bipolarity: clinical and treatment is-sues. Presented at the 156th annual meeting of the American Psychi-atric Association, San Francisco, CA, May 2003

McElroy SL, Strakowski SM, Keck PE Jr, et al: Differences and similari-ties in mixed and pure mania. Compr Psychiatry 36:187–194, 1995

Miller LJ: Use of electroconvulsive therapy during pregnancy. Hosp Community Psychiatry 45:444–450, 1994

Muller-Oerlinghausen B, Passoth PM, Poser W, et al: Effect of long-term treatment with neuroleptics or lithium salts on carbohydrate metab-olism. Amneimitteforschung 22:432–439, 1978

Newport DJ, Hostetter A, Arnold A, et al: The treatment of postpartum depression: minimizing infant exposures. J Clin Psychiatry 63 (suppl 7):31–44, 2002

O'Donovan, Kusumakar V, Graves GR, et al: Menstrual abnormalities and polycystic ovary syndrome in women taking valproate for bipo-lar disorder. J Clin Psychiatry 63:322–330, 2002

O'Hara MW, Stuart S, Gorman LL, et al: Efficacy of interpersonal psy-chotherapy for postpartum depression. Arch Gen Psychiatry 57:1039–1045, 2000

Omtzigt JG, Los FJ, Grobbee DE, et al: The risk of spina bifida aperta af-ter first-trimester exposure to valproate in a prenatal cohort. Neurol-ogy 42 (suppl 5):119–125, 1992

Pasquali R, Cassimirri E: The impact of obesity on hyperandrogenism and polycystic ovary syndrome in premenopausal women. Clin Endocrinol 39:1–16, 1993

Patten SB, Lamarre CJ: Can drug-induced depressions be identified by their clinical features? Can J Psychiatry 37:213–215, 1992

Paykel ES, Mueller PS, De La Vergne PM: Amitriptyline weight gain and carbohydrate craving. Br J Psychiatry 123:501–507, 1973

Pearlstein T, Steiner M: Non-antidepressant treatment of premenstrual syndrome. J Clin Psychiatry 61 (suppl 12):22–27, 2000

Perugi G, Musetti L, Simonini E, et al: Gender-mediated clinical features of depressive illness: the importance of temperamental differences. Br J Psychiatry 157:835–841, 1990

Petho B, Karczag I, Czeizel A: Family accumulated schizophrenia (folie a sinq) in association with Stein Leventhal syndrome. Psychiatr Clin North Am 15:206–211, 1982

Physicians' Desk Reference, 58th Edition. Montvale, NJ, Thomson Healthcare, 2004

Pierpoint T, McKeigue PM, Issacs AJ, et al: Mortality of women with polycystic ovary syndrome at long term follow up. J Clin Epidemiol 51:581–586, 1998

Pi–Sunyer FX: Health implications in obesity. Am J Clin Nutr 53:1595S–16035, 1991

Price WA, DiMarzio L: Premenstrual tension syndrome in rapid-cycling bipolar affective disorder. J Clin Psychiatry 47:415–417, 1986

Price WA, Giannini AJ: Antidepressant effects of estrogen. J Clin Psychiatry 46:506, 1985

Price WA, Giannini AJ, Seng CS: Use of L–tryptophan in the treatment of premenstrual tension: a case report. Psychiatry Forum 13:44–46, 1985

Printz DJ, Das A, Stricks LS, et al: Menstrual cycle phase and mood in bipolar disorder. Presented at the 154th annual meeting of the American Psychiatric Association, New Orleans, Louisiana, May 2001

Rapkin AJ, Mikacich JA, Moatakef-Imani B, et al: The clinical nature and formal diagnosis of premenstrual, postpartum, and perimenopausal affective disorders. Curr Psychiatry Rep 4:419–428, 2002

Rasgon NL, Altshuler LL, Gudeman D, et al: Medication status and polycystic ovary syndrome in women with bipolar disorder: a preliminary report. J Clin Psychiatry 61:173–178, 2000

Rasgon N, Bauer M, Glenn T, et al: Gender differences on mood patterns in bipolar disorder. Presented at the 155th annual meeting of the American Psychiatric Association, Philadelphia, PA, May 2002

Rasgon N, Bauer M, Glenn T, et al: Menstrual cycle related mood changes in women with bipolar disorder. Bipolar Disord 5:48–52, 2003

Regier DA, Narrow WE, Rae DS, et al: The de facto U.S. mental and addictive disorders service system: epidemiologic catchment area prospective 1-year prevalence rates of disorders and services. Arch Gen Psychiatry 50:85–94, 1993

Robb JC, Young LT, Cooke RG, et al: Gender differences in patients with bipolar disorder influence outcome in the medical outcomes survey (SF-20) subscale scores. J Affect Disord 49:189–193, 1998

Rosa FW: Spina bifida in infants of women treated with carbamazepine during pregnancy. N Engl J Med 324:674–677, 1991

Rubinow DR: Psychiatric disorders of the late luteal phase, in Psychopharmacology in Practice: Clinical and Research Update 1995. Bethesda, MD, The Foundation for Advanced Education in the Sciences, 1995, pp 155–183

Rubinow DR, Hoban MC, Grover GN, et al: Changes in plasma hormones across the menstrual cycle in patients with menstrually related mood disorder and in control subjects. Am J Obstet Gynecol 158:5–11, 1988

Rush AJ, Giles DE, Schlesser MA, et al: Dexamethasone response, thyrotropin-releasing hormone stimulation, rapid eye movement latency, and subtypes of depression. Biol Psychiatry 41:915–928, 1997

Rybakowski JK, Twardowska K: The dexamethasone/corticotropin-releasing hormone test in depression in bipolar and unipolar affective illness. J Psychiatr Res 33:363–370, 1999

Sabers A, Buchholt JM, Uldall P, et al: Lamotrigine plasma levels reduced by oral contraceptives. Epilepsy Res 47:151–154, 2001

Saltar N, Tan CE, Han TS, et al: Associations of indices of adiposity with atherogenic lipoprotein subfractions. Int J Obes Relat Metab Disord 22:432–439, 1998

Sassi RB, Nicoletti M, Brambilla P, et al: Decreased pituitary volume in patients with bipolar disorder. Biol Psychiatry 50:271–280, 2001

Schmider J, Lammers CH, Gotthardt U, et al: Combined dexamethasone/corticotropin-releasing hormone test in acute and remitted manic patients, in acute depression, and in normal controls, I. Biol Psychiatry 38:797–802, 1995

Schmidt PJ, Grover GN, Hoban MC, et al: State dependent alterations in the perception of life events in menstrual related mood disorders. Am J Psychiatry 147:230–234, 1990

Schmidt PJ, Nieman LK, Grover GN, et al: Lack of effect of induced menses on symptoms in women with premenstrual syndrome. N Engl J Med 324:1174–1179, 1991

Schmidt PJ, Roca CA, Bloch M, et al: The perimenopause and affective disorders. Semin Reprod Endocrinol 15:91–100, 1997

Silverstone T, Smith G, Goodall E: Prevalence of obesity in patients receiving depot antipsychotics. Br J Psychiatry 153:214–217, 1988

Solomon CG, Hu FB, Dunaif A, et al: Long or highly irregular menstrual cycles as a marker for risk of type 2 diabetes mellitus. JAMA 286:2421–2426, 2001

Solomon DA, Keitner GI, Miller IW, et al: Course of illness and maintenance treatment for patients with bipolar disorder. J Clin Psychiatry 56:5–13, 1995

Spinelli MG: Interpersonal psychotherapy for depressed antepartum women: a pilot study. Am J Psychiatry 154:1028–1030, 1997

Taylor MA, Abrams R: Gender differences in bipolar affective disorder. J Affect Disord 3:261–271, 1981

Thakore JH, Dinan TG: Blunted dexamethasone-induced growth hormone responses in acute mania. Psychoneuroendocrinology 21:695–701, 1996

Thakore JH, O'Keane V, Dinan TG: d-Fenfluramine-induced prolactin responses in mania: evidence for serotonergic subsensitivity. Am J Psychiatry 153:1460–1463, 1996

Tondo L, Baldessarini RJ: Rapid cycling in women and men with bipolar manic-depressive disorders. Am J Psychiatry 155:1434–1436, 1998

Vajda F, Lander C, O'Brien T, et al: Australian pregnancy registry of women taking antiepileptic drugs. Epilepsia 45(11):1466, 2004

VanPraag HM: Management of depression with serotonin precursors. Biol Psychiatry 16:291–309, 1981

Vestergaard P, Poulstrup I, Schou M: Prospective studies on a lithium cohort, 3: tremor, weight gain, diarrhea, psychological complaints. Acta Psychiatry Scand 78:434–441, 1988

Viguera AC, Nonacs R, Cohen LS, et al: Risk of recurrence of bipolar disorder in pregnant and nonpregnant women after discontinuing lithium maintenance. Am J Psychiatry 157:179–184, 2000a

Viguera AC, Tondo L, Baldessarini RJ: Sex differences in response to lithium treatment. Am J Psychiatry 157:1509–1511, 2000b

Viguera AC, Cohen LS, Baldessarini RJ, et al: Managing bipolar disorder during pregnancy: weighing the risks and benefits. Can J Psychiatry 47:426–436, 2002a

Viguera AC, Cohen LS, Reminick A, et al: Risk of recurrence among pregnant women with bipolar disorder. Presented at the 155th annual meeting of the American Psychiatric Association, Philadelphia, PA, May 2002b

Wehr TA: Causes and treatments of rapid cycling affective disorder, in Pharmacotherapy of Depression: Applications for the Outpatient Practitioner. Edited by Amsterdam J. New York, Marcel Dekker, 1990, pp 401–426

Wehr TA, Sack DA, Rosenthal NE, et al: Rapid cycling affective disorder: contributing factors and treatment responses in 51 patients. Am J Psychiatry 145:179–184, 1988

Weintraub M, Rubio A, Golik A, et al: Sibutramine in weight control: a dose-ranging, efficacy study. Clin Pharmacol Ther 50:330–337, 1991

Wisner KL, Peindl KS, Perel JM, et al: Verapamil treatment for women with bipolar disorder. Biol Psychiatry 51:745–752, 2002

Yang YS, Nowakowska C, Becker OV, et al: Weight loss during the first two months of open adjunctive zonisamide for obesity in bipolar disorders patients. Presented at the 156th annual meeting of the American Psychiatric Association, San Francisco, CA, May 2003

Yen SSC: Chronic anovulation caused by peripheral endocrine disorders, in Reproductive Endocrinology: Physiology, Pathophysiology and Clinical Management, 3rd Edition. Edited by Yen SSC, Jaffe RB. Philadelphia, PA, WB Saunders, 1991, pp 576–630

Index

*Page numbers printed in **boldface** refer to tables or figures*